Heart
healthy
for life

READER'S DIGEST

Published by
The Reader's Digest Association Limited
London • New York • Sydney • Montreal

Heart
healthy
for life

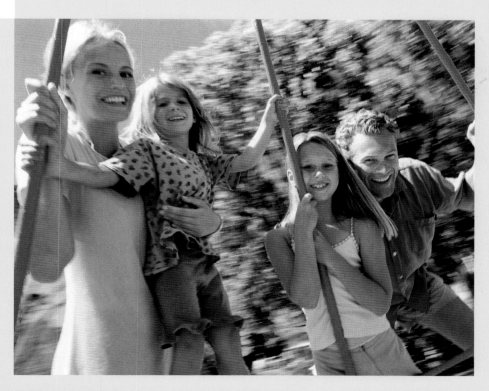

The ultimate guide to preventing and even reversing heart disease

READER'S DIGEST
Project Staff

Medical consultants
Dr John Cormack BDS MB BS MRCS LRCP
Dr Rajesh Aggarwal MD FRCP(Lond)

Project editor
Rachel Warren Chadd

Designer
Heather Dunleavy

Assistant editor
Jill Steed

Researcher
Angelika Romacker

Proofreader
Ron Pankhurst

Indexer
Marie Lorimer

READER'S DIGEST
General Books

Editorial director
Cortina Butler

Art director
Nick Clark

Executive editor
Julian Browne

Picture resource manager
Martin Smith

Pre-press account manager
Penelope Grose

Origination
Colour Systems Limited, London

Printing and binding
Cayfosa Quebecor, Barcelona, Spain

READER'S DIGEST USA

**Editor in chief and
publishing director**
Neil Wertheimer

Medical consultant
Rita F Redberg MD MSc
Associate Professor of Medicine,
  University of California
  San Francisco School of Medicine,
  Division of Cardiology

Writer
Peter Jaret

Design
Nina Scerbo Design Inc.

HEART HEALTHY FOR LIFE was originated by the
editorial team of The Reader's Digest Association, Inc.,
USA

This edition was adapted and published by
The Reader's Digest Association Limited
11 Westferry Circus, Canary Wharf
London E14 4HE

We are committed to both the quality of our products
and the service we provide to our customers. We value
your comments, so please feel free to contact us on
08705 113366 or via our website at:
www.readersdigest.co.uk
If you have any comments or suggestions about
the content of our books, email us at:
gbeditorial@readersdigest.co.uk

Note to Readers

While the creators of this work have made every effort
to be as accurate and up to date as possible, medical
and pharmacological knowledge is constantly changing.
Readers are recommended to consult a qualified medical
specialist for individual advice. The writers, researchers,
editors and publishers of this work cannot be held liable for
any errors and omissions, or actions that may be taken as a
consequence of information contained within this work.

About this book

Barbara Harpham
National Director, National Heart Research Fund

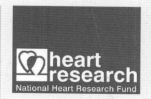

In recent years astonishing breakthroughs have been achieved in the battle against heart disease. But the journey is far from over; heart disease is still Britain's biggest killer. At Heart Research we promote its prevention, treatment and cure through grants to hospitals and universities throughout the UK. Many things now taken for granted, such as heart valves, angioplasty and, more recently, amazing artificial heart pumps, would simply not have been developed when they were without our help. We also realize that healthy living plays a vital role in combating heart disease. That's why we consider the strategies set out in **Heart Healthy for Life** present some of the best ways available to protect yourself and your family.

What is a healthy lifestyle? In an age when we are bombarded with conflicting facts about what to eat and how to exercise, it's difficult to make the right choices. Here, at last, is a book that will show you how to make changes that can protect your heart and give you a better quality of life. Its key message is one that Heart Research itself advocates in its healthy lifestyles programme to schools, businesses and community groups nationwide. By explaining exactly how bad habits can dramatically increase your risk of heart disease, we have helped to convince numerous people that changing just a few of them is well worth the effort. Too much fatty food, too little exercise, too much stress and smoking are all likely to lead to trouble – especially if you have risk factors such as high blood pressure, raised cholesterol or a family history of heart attacks.

In similar fashion, **Heart Healthy for Life** offers a wealth of practical, preventive strategies. Put them into practice and – as research has shown – you could add years to your life. This book sets you on the right path: it's your choice to do all you can to ensure that your life is longer, healthier and more enjoyable.

Foreword

Dr Rajesh Aggarwal

Consultant cardiologist, Basildon & Thurrock University Hospitals, NHS Foundation Trust

Our ability to diagnose and treat coronary heart disease (CHD) has improved out of all recognition in the 15 years since I qualified as a doctor. Despite the enormous advances, however, it remains a major threat in the UK, claiming the lives of one in four men and one in five women – some 140,000 deaths annually. In addition, the escalating costs of treating coronary heart disease place a huge burden on the NHS and the nation's economy.

Yet much can be done to prevent and treat CHD. Advances in drug treatment and technology alike have made us better at dealing with heart attack, angina and heart failure – all consequences of blocked coronary arteries. Among the most important advances are the developments in stent technology; stents are expandable metal-mesh tubes surgically implanted to keep an unblocked artery open. The latest 'smart' stents are impregnated with drugs which leach out slowly and can dramatically reduce the recurrence of blockages.

Much progress has also been made in the use of drugs to reduce the risk of further problems in heart attack victims; 'statins' for lowering cholesterol and good old aspirin for reducing blood stickiness are now acknowledged as some of the most effective therapies available. Death rates in patients with heart failure can also be cut substantially by using simple, commonly available drugs known as beta-blockers and ACE inhibitors. But people affected by heart disease also need to know and understand what therapies and drugs are available to help them – something which this book clearly explains – in order to take charge of their own condition.

So much can be done to prevent heart disease taking hold in the first place and **Heart Healthy for Life** provides extremely useful strategies. For instance, the most important reversible risk factor for developing blockages in coronary arteries is smoking. This book provides a sensible and effective stop smoking plan. We could all take more exercise than we do and pay attention to our diet – in particular our intake of saturated fat and salt – and here you'll find valuable tips that will help you to achieve these objectives.

> " So much can be done to prevent heart disease taking hold in the first place and Heart Healthy for Life provides extremely useful strategies. "

People who are at particular risk of developing heart disease, such as those with diabetes or with a close relative who has suffered heart disease at a young age, should pay particular attention to these issues and should also have their blood pressure checked regularly and their cholesterol measured. High blood pressure and raised cholesterol are both associated with an increased risk of coronary heart disease and much can be done to lower both of them without immediately resorting to drug treatment.

After undergoing a treadmill exercise test as part of a medical check-up, one of my patients, an eminent businessman, was shocked to learn that he might have angina. He worked 14 hours a day, was overweight, smoked and took no regular physical exercise; he was also found to have high blood pressure and elevated blood cholesterol. A coronary angiogram (X-ray dye test) showed blockages in all three of his heart arteries and he reluctantly accepted the need to undergo coronary artery bypass surgery.

The operation went well and his recovery was aided by enrolment into a cardiac rehabilitation programme. He accepted the advice he was given. He stopped smoking, lost more than 3 stone (20kg) and installed a mini-gym in his home. He continues to run his extremely successful business but now exercises for 45 minutes daily and has set up a weight and blood pressure club at his workplace, which has been warmly welcomed by his colleagues.

Many of my patients, like this man, are shocked by the initial diagnosis of heart disease and some even go through a phase of denial. But with help and advice from their healthcare professionals and the sort of strategies advocated in **Heart Healthy for Life**, most feel empowered to take charge of their condition and modify their lifestyle accordingly. The end result is patients who not only feel better but also have more zest for life and greater confidence in the future.

It takes a great deal of commitment and willpower to embark on lifestyle changes which are heart healthy. This book will help to convince you of the need to make these changes and the potential benefits you will reap.

Contents

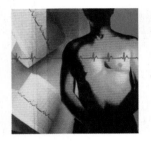
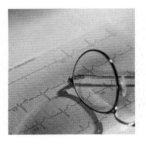
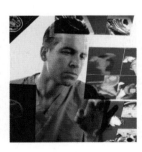
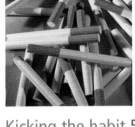
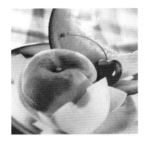
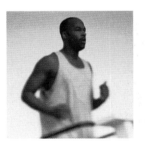

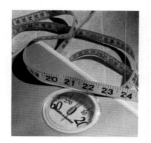

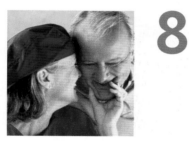
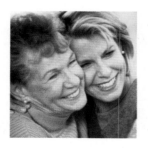
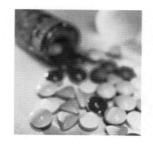
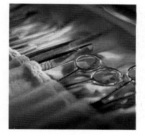
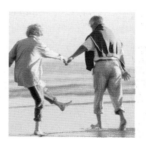

1

The heart
of the matter

First, it's time for some self-congratulation. Since the 1950s, health experts have sounded the alarm about a rising epidemic of heart disease among Britons. But death rates from heart disease have been falling steadily since the 1970s – for the under 65s by a staggering 44 per cent. According to the British Heart Foundation, the death rate from cardiovascular disease fell by 39 per cent for men and 41 per cent for women, between 1989 and 1999.

However, there is no room for complacency. Despite the progress we have made, cardiovascular disease remains the single most serious health threat that Britons face. More people in the UK die of it today than any other illness. Cardiovascular disease, which includes diseases of the heart or blood vessels, killed some 117,500 people in 2002 – that was 322 deaths every day.

According to the British Heart Foundation, about 2.7 million people in the UK suffer from some form of cardiovascular disease; almost one in eight people have been diagnosed with a disease of the heart or circulatory system. Despite the fall in the overall death rate – which has been put down to better treatment and improved lifestyles – more people are developing heart disease.

But there's good news, too. Heart disease isn't inevitable. In fact, it is one of the most preventable of all serious illnesses.

You're in control

By making a few simple changes to your daily routine, you can dramatically reduce your risk of heart attack. And you don't have to turn your life upside down to do it. Take a brisk walk after dinner in place of watching one sitcom on most nights of the week, and you've already started to arm yourself against trouble. Trim a bit of saturated fat from your menu, and you'll compound that protection. If you smoke, muster the courage to quit and you'll halve your risk of heart disease.

There's plenty your doctor can do, too. Thanks to advances in treatment, the prospects of living a long and active life even if you've been diagnosed with advanced heart disease are better than

> "Despite the progress we have made, cardiovascular disease remains the single most serious health threat that Britons face."

ever before. New medications can lower elevated cholesterol and high blood pressure, helping to keep heart attacks and strokes at bay. Sophisticated surgical techniques are clearing blocked arteries and repairing damage to the heart itself.

We know more today than even 10 years ago about what keeps a heart healthy, what causes damage and how to avoid or repair that damage. *Heart Healthy for Life* will arm you with the latest medical findings and put this knowledge in your hands.

Your heart, in health and in sickness

The human heart beats an average of 70 times a minute, 4,200 times an hour, 100,800 times a day. With each beat, this muscular pump pushes blood through a complex network of blood vessels that, if laid end to end, would stretch 60,000 miles. Clearly, the heart is a pretty tough organ. Yet plenty of things can go wrong.

Progress on many fronts

What explains the dramatic decline in heart disease rates over the past 30 years? Surprisingly, researchers aren't sure. So much progress has been made in so many areas of heart disease prevention that it's likely that many changes have contributed. Still, it's important for researchers to know what works and what doesn't in order to focus public health efforts. Not long ago, scientists from the Harvard School of Public Health analysed a decade's worth of heart disease data from around the country. They estimated that 25 per cent of the decline in

coronary artery disease resulted from primary prevention efforts geared to keep healthy people from developing heart problems, such as the push to lower the amount of saturated fat in our diets. An additional 29 per cent was explained by secondary prevention efforts, those aimed at reducing risk factors such as high blood pressure and elevated cholesterol in people already diagnosed with heart trouble. And 43 per cent was attributed to advances in treatments, such as bypass surgery and techniques to repair blocked arteries.

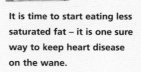

It is time to start eating less saturated fat – it is one sure way to keep heart disease on the wane.

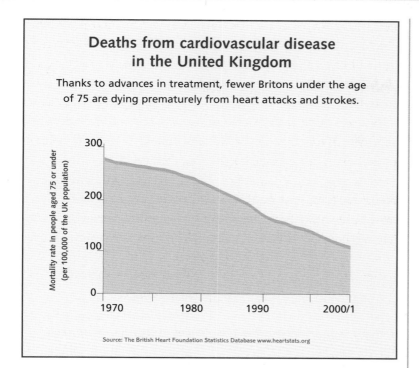

Deaths from cardiovascular disease in the United Kingdom

Thanks to advances in treatment, fewer Britons under the age of 75 are dying prematurely from heart attacks and strokes.

Mortality rate in people aged 75 or under (per 100,000 of the UK population)

300

200

100

0

1970   1980   1990   2000/1

Source: The British Heart Foundation Statistics Database www.heartstats.org

Heart disease takes many forms, from congenital defects in heart valves to infections that damage heart muscles. Far and away the greatest threat comes from a process called atherosclerosis, also known as hardening of the arteries. The chief culprit is cholesterol, a waxy substance that circulates through the blood.

Over time, cholesterol can build up to form deposits inside blood vessel walls. Like sediment in water pipes, these deposits may restrict blood flow. Eventually blockages can form. When the coronary arteries, which supply blood to the heart, become obstructed, the result is coronary artery disease, the leading cause of heart attacks. When vessels in the neck that supply blood to the brain narrow, carotid artery disease results. If the blockage becomes bad enough, portions of the brain can be robbed of the blood and oxygen they need, causing a stroke.

Too much of a good thing

Here's more proof that heart disease isn't inevitable: a century ago heart attacks were uncommon in many parts of the world. Even today, rates of heart disease vary widely from country to country. Why has cardiovascular disease become the number one killer in the United Kingdom? In a sense, we are the victims of our own good fortune. Labour-saving devices have taken over most hard physical work.

FAST FACT
In the United Kingdom, 30 per cent of deaths from coronary heart disease are related to unhealthy diets.

Food manufacturers have filled our tables with an array of tempting choices. At the same time, the demands of modern life seem to cause unprecedented pressure. This combination of abundant food (much of it laden with fat and salt), sedentary lifestyles and unrelenting stress can spell big trouble for our hearts.

Because cardiovascular disease is associated with rich diets and sedentary living, it has been called a disease of affluence. That is misleading. The risk is higher in many industrialized societies than in some less developed societies, partly because traditional diets are often much healthier than diets centred on processed foods. But in the UK, heart disease strikes at every level and in many respects the lower socio-economic groups are more at risk.

▼ Key finding

Adopting some new habits really can save your life, according to recent results from the Nurses' Health Study in the USA. Of more than 84,000 nurses, those who didn't smoke, who followed a heart healthy diet and exercised regularly were 80 per cent less likely than those with less healthy lifestyles to have a heart attack during a 14-year period of study.

The heart healthy approach

Heart Healthy for Life offers an action plan that will shore up your heart and circulatory system against future problems and even reverse some of the signs and symptoms of heart disease. It is worth the effort because research shows that making five lifestyle changes could prevent as many as four out of five cases of coronary artery disease. The same five changes will keep you healthier if you've already been diagnosed with heart problems. This is what will make all the difference:

1 **Kick the habit** If you smoke, this book will join the chorus of voices encouraging you to quit – and will show you how. Smoking is deadly for many reasons. Chemicals in cigarette smoke restrict the flow of blood and make blood cells called platelets stickier than normal, increasing the risk of a dangerous blood clot. Carbon monoxide from cigarette smoke reduces the amount of oxygen that reaches your heart. Give up, and you'll start reaping the health benefits from the moment you do.

2 **Get moving** Believe it or not, being a couch potato can be every bit as dangerous to your heart as smoking. If your idea of exercise is reaching for the remote control, don't worry. Becoming even moderately active – nothing more strenuous than 30 minutes of brisk walking most days of the week – could slash your chances of

Studying heart disease for decades

'In 1948, we didn't pay much attention to what we were eating,' recalls Walter Sullivan, 87, a retired lawyer from Massachusetts, USA. 'My favourite breakfast was eggs and bacon. My wife, Katie, and I smoked. We never exercised.'

That year the Sullivans volunteered to participate in a bold medical experiment being organized in their hometown of Framingham. Alarmed by the growing epidemic of heart disease in the United States, scientists from the US Public Health Service recruited more than 5,000 healthy residents aged 30 to 60 from Framingham.

Every two years the volunteers received a careful medical examination and a battery of tests. By analysing the data, researchers hoped to find clues to the causes of heart disease.

The Framingham Heart Study has been running for more than half a century. More than 20,000 people have participated. The Sullivans (and now their children) still go for regular examinations. Thanks to them, the study has helped to make dozens of lifesaving discoveries. Here are some of them:

1957 High blood pressure and high cholesterol levels linked to heart disease risk

1961 Researchers coin the term 'risk factor'

1962 Cigarette smoking shown to increase risk of heart disease

1967 Physical activity found to lower cardiovascular disease risk

1970 High blood pressure linked to increased risk of stroke

1974 Diabetes linked to cardiovascular disease danger

1977 Experts describe the effects of triglycerides, low-density lipoproteins (LDL cholesterol) and high-density lipoproteins (HDL cholesterol) on heart disease risk

1981 Filter cigarettes shown to offer no protection against heart disease

1988 High levels of HDL cholesterol shown to reduce cardiovascular disease risk

1997 Researchers describe the cumulative effects of smoking, high blood pressure and high cholesterol on heart disease

1998 Discovery of gene linked to high blood pressure

Today, the researchers are investigating genetic links to heart disease and exploring other risk factors that may provide early warning signs of trouble.

These days, Walter Sullivan is much more careful about his diet, thanks to the findings he and his family helped to generate. 'Eggs are a special treat now. I eat more fish and less beef than before. Most days of the week I spend half an hour riding an exercise bicycle and working with free weights. And of course we gave up smoking a long time ago.' At 87 he still gardens in the spring, rakes leaves in autumn and shovels snow in the winter – a testament to the benefits of a heart-healthy lifestyle.

Top 5 causes of death in the UK

1 Heart disease
2 Cancer
3 Stroke
4 Respiratory diseases
5 Liver diseases

Source: Office of National Statistics
Figures for 2002

having a heart attack almost in half. We'll explain how buying a simple device called a step counter can spur your exercise efforts and keep you on track.

3 Eat well No, we don't mean sitting down to a meal of bean sprouts and lentils every night, or giving up the foods you love. Some of the world's most delicious cuisines – including Asian and Mediterranean diets – are also among the healthiest. By stealing a few of their secrets, you can guard your heart while satisfying your taste buds.

4 Slim down At any given moment, 25 per cent of adult Britons say they want to lose weight – with very good reason: high blood pressure, diabetes and elevated cholesterol are linked to being overweight. Being moderately overweight increases your risk of heart disease. Being obese, or seriously overweight, is more dangerous. If you've tried and failed to lose weight, don't be discouraged. Shedding even a few pounds can make a positive difference to your heart. We'll show you how to cut calories without going hungry. Plus we'll tell you how you can boost your metabolism to burn more calories all day long and keep the weight off – permanently.

5 Relax People who score high on tests that measure anger have been shown to run a higher risk of heart disease. And it's common for heart attacks to occur during stressful periods. Even if stress doesn't cause heart disease, a hectic day at the office or anxiety over problems at home can make it a lot harder for you to stick to your resolution to take that walk during your lunch hour or shun the chocolate bar tempting you. Learning a few techniques to defuse anger and stress can help.

And now for a change ...

Thanks to more than 50 years of research, doctors today know the prescription for a healthy heart. So why aren't more people following it?

The reason is simple: Change isn't always easy. Modifying the way you eat – even switching from semi-skimmed milk to skimmed, for example – requires a commitment. Something as seemingly feasible as walking 30 minutes a day on most days of the week can be difficult if you have a demanding schedule or you simply aren't used to exercising. And the prospect of quitting smoking can be downright daunting.

Eating for
a healthy
heart can be a
delicious endeavour.
Get ready for a treat.

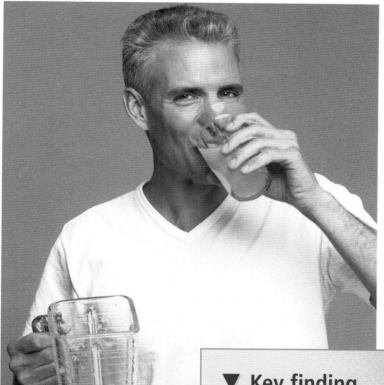

▼ Key finding

Do you want to clean up your arteries? US researchers at Stanford University, followed 300 volunteers, all of whom had atherosclerosis. Half received standard medical care. The other half were given a programme of intensive counselling on improving their diet, exercising and other heart-healthy lifestyles. Four years later, those who received the counselling had a 47 per cent lower rate of artery narrowing. The condition is not reversible but there is increasing evidence that lifestyle and medication can halt its progress.

But you *can* do it. Psychologists who study how people make changes have gained a better understanding of what it takes. In *Heart Healthy for Life*, we'll share many of their insights to help to smooth your way.

One crucial discovery is worth mentioning here. Whether you're trying to improve your diet, stop biting your fingernails or become more active, experts have discovered that the process of change takes place in stages. According to James O. Prochaska Ph.D., a professor of clinical and health psychology at the University of Rhode Island, there are five basic stages of change. If you're just beginning to think about tweaking your lifestyle to become heart healthy, for instance, you're

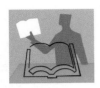

TERMS TO KNOW

ATHEROSCLEROSIS The medical term for hardening of the arteries, which is caused when deposits of fat, cholesterol and other substances reduce the flow of blood through arteries

CARDIOVASCULAR DISEASE Any disease that affects the heart or the blood vessels

CAROTID ARTERY DISEASE Blockage of the neck arteries that supply the brain

CHOLESTEROL A waxy substance that, in excessive amounts, can lead to atherosclerosis

CORONARY ARTERY DISEASE Blockage of the arteries that supply blood to the heart

HEART ATTACK (MYOCARDIAL INFARCTION) Damage to part of the heart muscle caused when a blockage in one of the coronary arteries robs heart tissue of blood and oxygen

PRIMARY PREVENTION Preventing the conditions that lead to heart disease, such as high blood pressure and elevated cholesterol

SECONDARY PREVENTION Preventing heart attacks or further cardiovascular damage in people already diagnosed with heart disease

STROKE Damage that occurs when an artery blockage robs the brain of blood and oxygen

at the 'contemplation' stage. If you've been trying to make some changes and haven't quite succeeded yet, you're at a stage called 'preparation'.

Why does it matter? Because knowing your current stage of change can help you to target strategies that will propel you to the next stage. Find out how ready you really are to get heart healthy by taking this short quiz. It examines just one aspect of your lifestyle – your diet. Circle the number beside the statement that most closely describes how you feel right now about making the changes in the way you eat that could lower your risk of heart disease – cutting back on saturated fat, for instance, and eating more fruit, vegetables and whole grains. Each of these statements corresponds to one of the five stages of change.

1. 'To be perfectly honest, I'm just not willing to change at this moment.' (precontemplation)
2. 'I sometimes think about trying to eat a healthier diet but I haven't actually done anything about changing it yet.' (contemplation)
3. 'I do try to eat more healthily now and then, but I just haven't been able to stick with it.' (preparation)
4. 'I recently began eating a healthier diet, and now my goal is to try to make my new habits stick.' (action)
5. 'I've been following a heart-healthy diet for six months or more already.' (maintenance)

The statement you choose indicates how far along the path you are to making sensible adjustments to your diet – one important step toward becoming heart healthy. Don't worry if you haven't come very far. Knowing where you stand now can help you to focus on what you need to do to move forward. On the next page you'll find some basic strategies tailored to each of the five stages.

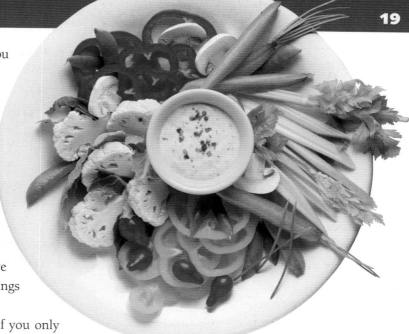

I Precontemplation If you are honestly not willing to change at this time, chances are you're not yet sure the benefits are worth the trouble. In *Heart Healthy for Life* we will persuade you that not only can adjusting your habits save your life, it will also make you feel better, look better and have more energy to do the things you enjoy.

2 Contemplation Even if you only think about making positive changes, that is already a step forward. At this stage, it's important to begin making some practical plans to turn your good intentions into actions, such as buying a low-fat cookbook or resolving to have an extra serving of vegetables at dinner.

3 Preparation If you've been trying to eat a healthier diet but have not had much success, take a look at the obstacles that have stopped you. Maybe you often have to grab lunch on the run – and

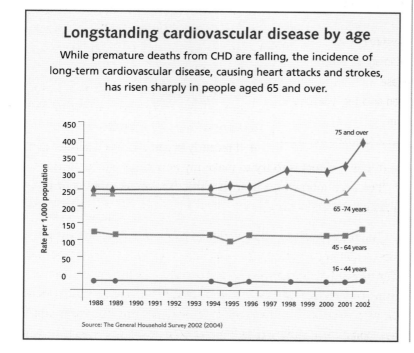

Longstanding cardiovascular disease by age

While premature deaths from CHD are falling, the incidence of long-term cardiovascular disease, causing heart attacks and strokes, has risen sharply in people aged 65 and over.

Source: The General Household Survey 2002 (2004)

5 MYTHS ABOUT HEART DISEASE

1 Only men have heart attacks.
Wrong. Heart disease is the leading cause of death for women, too.

2 If heart disease runs in your family, there's not much you can do.
Even someone with a family history of the disease can do plenty to prevent a heart attack.

3 Heart disease is inevitable later in life.
Not so. In some parts of the world, heart disease is uncommon even among very old people.

4 The biggest danger from cigarette smoking is lung cancer.
In fact, the largest proportion of deaths related to smoking is due to heart disease.

5 If your cholesterol is normal, you don't need to worry about heart disease.
Cholesterol is only one of several risk factors, including high blood pressure and family health history.

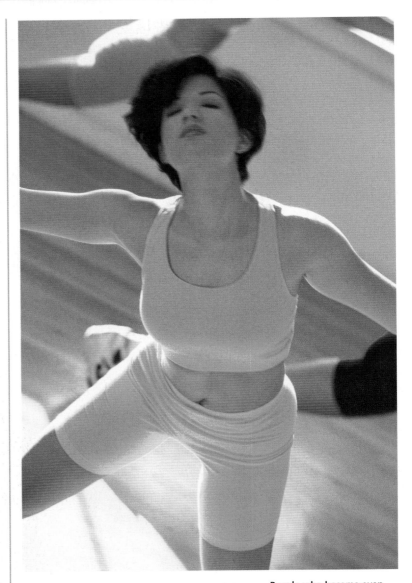

People who become even moderately active can cut their risk of heart disease by as much as half. If you already have heart disease, exercise can lower your risk of heart attack and stroke.

the only place to stop is a fast-food restaurant. Maybe you're doing fine until you dine out, and then you eat a lot more than you should. For each obstacle, think of a way around it – packing a lunch, for instance, or inviting a friend to come and share that gigantic plate of pasta at your favourite restaurant – that way you'll save money too!

4 Action You've already turned intent into action. For almost anyone who tries to make a lifestyle change, obstacles can appear, sometimes out of nowhere. Remind yourself that a small lapse doesn't mean you've fallen apart. Plan ahead with strategies for times when you may find it hard to stick with your goals (around holidays and festivities, for instance).

5 Maintenance If you've already reached stage 5, congratulations! You're well on your way to a heart-healthy life. At this stage, it's important to remind yourself of the many benefits you're reaping and to stick with the plan. In *Heart Healthy for Life* we'll give you tips on how to make your new habits last a lifetime.

Never too late – or too early

Younger adults tend to think they're invincible. The threat of problems like cancer or heart disease seems so distant that these people rarely take the risk seriously. On the other hand, older people sometimes think it's too late to make meaningful changes because the damage is already done.

Both groups are wrong. Autopsies performed on young adults, teenagers and even children, have often uncovered signs of fatty streaks in blood vessel walls – evidence that atherosclerosis has already begun. Children in the UK are also starting to show raised cholesterol levels. True, some may suffer from a genetic condition that causes unusually high cholesterol. But most of them have high cholesterol simply because they eat too much saturated fat. In a study at Dundee University, researchers found 20 per cent of teenagers had early signs of heart disease. It's never too early, in other words, to start taking care of your heart.

It's never too late, either. There's plenty of evidence that older people who make heart-healthy changes reap the benefits. A summary of trials performed in Europe shows a consistent 15 to 20 per cent improvement in heart failure patients who underwent a training programme of walking, cycling and exercise. There was significant improvement in survival and a reduction in hospital readmissions.

Researchers at the Cooper Institute for Aerobics Research in Dallas, Texas, found that older men who exercised and improved their overall fitness reduced their risk of dying over the five-year study period by 44 per cent. Even long-time smokers can reduce the heart-related damage caused by cigarettes if they stop smoking today.

So there's no better time than right now to take the first step toward a healthier heart – and *Heart Healthy for Life* will show you how.

> *Younger adults tend to think they're invincible. On the other hand, older people sometimes think it's too late to make meaningful changes.*

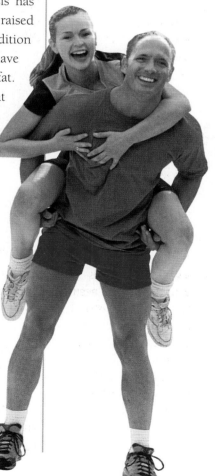

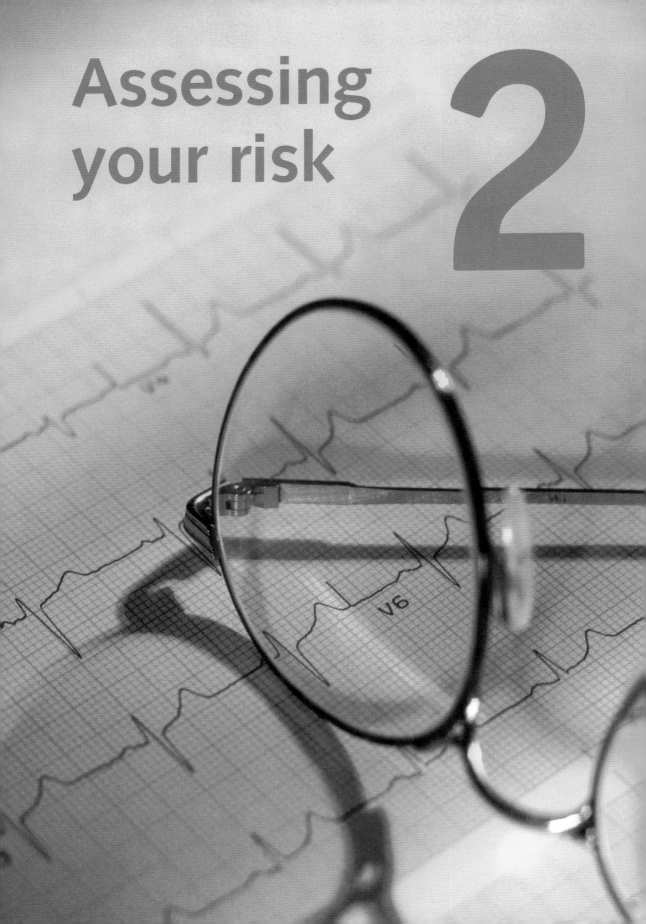

Assessing your risk

2

Fifty years ago, the cause of most heart attacks was a mystery. No one knew why they happened at all – let alone why they happened to some people and not others. Today, researchers understand many of the factors that put people in the path of danger. Knowing exactly how you rate in these areas will help you and your doctor to target a powerful prevention strategy tailored to your risk profile.

Some points against you, like a family history of heart disease, you simply have to accept. But by lessening the hazards under your control, like high blood pressure or high cholesterol, you can slash your risk of a heart attack or stroke. If you've already suffered either one of these, you can go a long way towards avoiding another.

An international detective story

When researchers first began to unravel the mystery of heart disease, they began with one tantalizing clue: the odd fact that the risk of heart attacks varied dramatically in different parts of the world. In Finland and the United States, for instance, heart disease topped the list of leading causes of death. In other places, like Greece, it was exceedingly rare.

In a now famous investigation called the Seven Countries Study, scientists back in the 1950s set out to discover why. They compared thousands of people in Japan, the United States, Greece, Italy, Finland, the former Yugoslavia and the Netherlands, using blood tests and questionnaires. One of their first discoveries was that cholesterol levels in the blood varied widely in different parts of the world. In addition, there seemed to be a close connection between these levels and the risk of heart attacks. The higher a person's cholesterol, the greater the danger.

Since then, researchers have identified a host of other factors that increase the risk of developing heart disease. Some are ones we can't alter and over which we have no control, such as our age, gender or family health history. Many more are things we can change. These include medical conditions (such as diabetes and high blood pressure) that, if left untreated, can damage arteries or

> "By lessening the hazards under your control, like high blood pressure or high cholesterol, you can slash your risk of a heart attack or stroke."

TERMS TO KNOW

BODY MASS INDEX (BMI)
A scale used to measure body mass. To see how you rate, divide your body weight in kilos by your height in metres squared. Or divide your weight in pounds by your height in inches squared and multiply the total by 703

CONGESTIVE HEART FAILURE A condition that occurs when the heart can no longer efficiently pump blood around the body, leading to a build-up of fluid in the lungs and body tissues

DIASTOLIC The bottom number of a blood pressure reading. Diastolic blood pressure is the lowest pressure that occurs when the heart relaxes between beats

FAMILIAL HYPERCHOLESTEROLAEMIA Inherited form of high cholesterol that greatly increases heart disease risk

HDL High-density lipoprotein, a beneficial component of cholesterol that promotes the breakdown and removal of artery-clogging cholesterol

HYPERTENSION High blood pressure

LDL Low-density lipoprotein, the dangerous component of cholesterol that can gather on the inside of blood vessels, forming deposits that block blood flow

SYSTOLIC The top number of a blood pressure reading. Systolic blood pressure is the highest pressure that occurs when the heart contracts with each heartbeat

TRIGLYCERIDES Fat particles in the blood; high levels of triglycerides can increase cardiovascular risk

weaken the heart. They also include lifestyle factors, such as exercise and diet, over which we do have control.

A word about risk

Having one or more risk factors for heart disease doesn't mean you're doomed to have a heart attack. Think about seat belts. Driving without a seat belt increases your chances of being severely injured or dying in a crash. Of course, some people who don't use seat belts will never be in an accident, and some who do may be hurt or killed in a car. But overall, the risks are much greater if you don't wear seat belts than if you do.

The same goes for heart disease. Just as not wearing a seat belt increases your chances of being injured in an accident, raised cholesterol or high blood pressure increases the odds on having heart problems later on. Eliminating or lessening such a risk can dramatically lower the hazard.

What if you don't have any risk factors? Are you safe from ever having a heart attack? Not entirely. For, while you're significantly less likely to develop heart disease, some heart attacks occur out of the blue, in the absence of any known risk factors. Why remains a mystery.

But one thing is clear: increasing the amount of exercise you do, choosing to eat more heart-protective foods and learning to put stress in its place are sensible moves, even if you aren't in any imminent danger. Think of them as an insurance policy against heart problems and all kinds of other illnesses, including diabetes and many types of cancer.

Risk factors you can't change

It may seem odd to worry about things you can't change. But recognizing your risk factors is essential to knowing your overall probability of developing heart disease in the next ten years. Plus, it creates real incentive to take charge of what you can change. Here are the main risks you may be stuck with.

I **Inherited risk** If heart disease runs in your family – especially heart attacks that occur before the age of 50 for men and 55 for women – you're likely to be at increased risk. The most significant threat is associated with an inherited condition called familial hypercholesterolaemia, which causes dangerously high cholesterol levels as high as 8.9mmol/l (millimoles per litre) when the healthy target is 5mmol/l. A tendency toward high blood pressure, obesity or diabetes can also be inherited.

Does a family history of early heart disease mean you're fated to have it, too? Not at all. But knowing your family history will help you and your doctor target the wisest prevention strategy. If you have hypercholesterolaemia, for instance, your doctor is likely to recommend changes in your diet and/or prescribe medications to bring your cholesterol level down and keep it down.

2 **Gender** More men than women develop cardiovascular disease. Men also develop it about a decade earlier than women do. Researchers don't know exactly why premenopausal women are protected, although oestrogen may play a role. After menopause, as

FAST FACT
According to the Blood Pressure Association, more than 120,000 people each year could be saved from suffering a stroke or heart attack if their blood pressure were better controlled.

'White coat' hypertension

Blood pressure usually rises when people are nervous or under stress. For some patients, ironically, one place that causes stress – and raises blood pressure – is a doctor's surgery, resulting in a phenomenon dubbed 'white coat' hypertension. You may be able to avoid this anomaly by sitting quietly in a chair for at least five minutes before the reading is taken with your arm at heart level. If you want to buy a blood pressure monitor to use at home, you should buy an upper arm model as these tend to give a more accurate reading. The British Hypertension Society has compiled a list of well-tested models, priced from around £55 to £115. Details are on their web site at: www.bpassoc.org.uk/information/information.htm

oestrogen levels decline, a woman's risk begins to rise. As men and women reach their 60s and 70s, the gender gap narrows. In the end, 47 per cent of all fatal heart attacks occur in women.

3 **Age** Risk increases with age. Half of all heart attacks in the United Kingdom occur in people over 65. That doesn't mean that cardiovascular disease is an inevitable part of ageing, however. In some parts of the world, it remains far less common at any age than it is here. A lifetime of healthy eating and plenty of physical activity can protect most people throughout their lives.

Risk factors you can change

The risk factors you can change far outnumber those you can't. That's good news. It means that even if you have a family history of heart disease you can make a huge dent in your inherited risk. Factors you can change come in two categories: medical conditions that contribute to heart disease and habits that affect your heart.

Medical conditions

I **High blood pressure** To supply oxygen and nutrients to every part of the body, your heart must pump with enough force, or pressure, to keep blood moving. When blood flow becomes restricted in the smaller branches of the arteries, the pressure has to be increased in order to push the blood through. (It is similar to what happens when you put your finger over the end of a garden hose. As you restrict the flow of water, the pressure increases.) The result is high blood pressure, also known as hypertension. This condition puts a strain on the blood vessels and on the heart. If left

▼ Key finding

Even blood pressure in the high-normal range (130-139/85-89) may be too high, according to a 2001 report from researchers involved in the Framingham Heart Study (see page 15). Comparing people with optimal blood pressure (under 120/80), those with even slightly elevated numbers were found to be twice as likely to develop cardiovascular disease. Blood pressure in the high-normal range was found to be particularly dangerous for women.

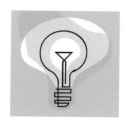

ASK THE EXPERT

'How can some cholesterol be good and some bad?'

James Cleeman MD, director of the US National Cholesterol Education Program:

'The difference between "good" and "bad" cholesterol is really the difference in the direction cholesterol is travelling in the blood: into the tissues of the body, where it can accumulate inside artery walls, or back to the liver, where it is eliminated.

First, a word about cholesterol. All cholesterol in the blood takes the form of small packets called lipoproteins, made up of fat (also called lipids) and protein. Just as oil and water don't mix, fat and blood don't mix. So lipoproteins are constructed with the fat on the inside and the protein molecules on the outside, allowing them to travel easily through the blood.

Low-density lipoprotein, or LDL (the so-called "bad" cholesterol), is cholesterol on its way into the tissues of the body, including artery walls. Too much of it can build up to create plaques on the lining of blood vessels. Blood clots can attach themselves to these plaques,

cutting off blood flow and causing a heart attack. In contrast, high-density lipoprotein, or HDL (the so-called "good" cholesterol), is cholesterol being carried away from the tissues to the liver for disposal.

It makes good sense, of course, to want to keep your levels of LDL low and your HDL high. In fact, we have very solid evidence that lowering your LDL levels will reduce heart attack risk. We have less evidence that raising HDL levels will bring down the danger, although most researchers are pretty sure it will. As it happens, we're much better at lowering LDL – through dietary changes or medication – than we are at raising HDL.

There are certainly ways to bring HDL numbers up – by increasing physical activity, for instance, and quitting smoking – and this is very important to heart health. But reducing LDL levels should be the prime focus of our efforts.'

untreated, it can inflate your odds of developing coronary artery disease by as much as three times and your chances of having a stroke by seven times.

These numbers are all the more worrying because as many as 16 million people in the UK suffer from high blood pressure. And most people don't even know they have it. High blood pressure is sometimes called a silent killer because it has no symptoms. The only way to diagnose it is to have your blood pressure tested. Adults should have their blood pressure measured every five years until the age of 80 – and every year, if it is high or high-normal.

What the numbers mean

BLOOD PRESSURE

Blood pressure is measured in millimeters of mercury, or mmHg. It includes two numbers, usually written as a fraction. The top number represents systolic blood pressure, or the highest pressure that occurs when your heart is contracting. The bottom number represents diastolic blood pressure, or the lowest pressure that occurs when your heart is relaxing and filling with blood.

The average healthy person has a blood pressure below 130/85. A reading of 120/80 or below is optimal. Anything above 140/90 is considered abnormal and is called high blood pressure or hypertension.

CHOLESTEROL

Until recently, most blood tests for cholesterol measured only total cholesterol. Now most doctors are aware that low-density lipoprotein, or LDL, is especially harmful to arteries and that high-density lipoprotein, or HDL, actually keeps arteries clear by removing the bad form. Therefore tests now compare levels of HDL and LDL, so that doctors can get a fairly reliable picture of your risk of heart disease. Your cholesterol screening results can also help your doctor to advise you on the best way to improve your cholesterol profile and lower your heart disease risk. In the UK cholesterol is measured in millimoles per litre, often abbreviated as mmol/l. There are no set targets for cholesterol levels in England and Wales, but experts generally agree that the following levels should be aimed for:

- Total cholesterol: no more than 5mmol/l
- HDL cholesterol: more than 1.15mmol/l
- LDL cholesterol: less than 3mmol/l

However, the average total cholesterol level in the UK is 5.8mmol/l – over the limit.

TRIGLYCERIDES

Cholesterol tests also typically measure the level of triglyceride, the other major fat, in the blood. Many studies have shown a strong connection between elevated triglyceride levels and increased risk of heart disease – although the link isn't as strong as that for cholesterol or high blood pressure. One reason is that triglyceride levels vary widely from person to person. Men tend to have higher levels than women. What's more, there is no evidence that high levels actually cause heart disease (unlike cholesterol, which plays a key role). Still, your doctor may want to know your levels in order to fine-tune your prescription for lowering your heart attack risk.

Triglyceride levels below 2mmol/l are considered healthy; a reading higher than 2mmol/l indicates increased risk. Fortunately, the same lifestyle changes that can lower your cholesterol will also improve your triglyceride levels. Losing weight may be especially important, as elevated triglyceride levels are associated with obesity.

2 High cholesterol The higher your total cholesterol, the greater your danger of cardiovascular disease. In the Framingham Heart Study, researchers found that people with a total cholesterol of 7.8mmol/l were twice as likely to develop heart disease as people with just under 4mmol/l. In another, more recent American study, the Multiple Risk Factor Intervention Trial, high cholesterol seemed to be an even greater risk factor. Of the 360,000 American men studied, those whose total cholesterol was above 7.8mmol/l were four times more likely to die of heart disease during the study than men with numbers below 4.7mmol/l.

What's wrong with having very high levels of cholesterol? The form of the waxy substance known as low-density lipoprotein, or LDL cholesterol, can build up inside artery walls, causing accumulations called plaques. These plaques lead to atherosclerosis (hardening of the arteries) and may eventually cause heart attacks or strokes. But there are many ways that people can bring down high LDL cholesterol, from cutting back on saturated fat and eating more fruit and vegetables to taking one of the new generation of cholesterol-lowering medications.

LDL isn't the whole story. Scientists now know that high density lipoprotein, or HDL – sometimes called 'good' cholesterol – is also important. HDL helps to remove damaging cholesterol from the blood, through the action of the liver. So the higher your level of this form of cholesterol, the lower your danger of clogged arteries and heart attacks.

For more information on the functions of LDL and HDL, see 'Ask the expert' on page 27, where the differences are explained in more detail.

3 Diabetes Diabetes impairs the body's ability to process sugar for energy. Your body normally converts some of the food you eat into glucose, a type of sugar. The hormone called insulin allows glucose to enter cells, where it is used for energy. Two forms of diabetes can disrupt this finely calibrated system. Type 1 diabetes occurs when the pancreas fails to produce enough insulin to process glucose. Type 2 diabetes, also called adult-onset diabetes, occurs when cells stop responding normally to insulin. If you have either one, your risk of cardiovascular disease is roughly twice that of the general population. Fortunately, for most people, medications and lifestyle changes can keep diabetes from threatening your heart or causing a stroke. For further information see the website of Diabetes UK: www.diabetes.org.uk

FAST FACT
As many as one million people with diabetes, in the UK, don't know they have the condition, which can, at least, double the risk of heart disease.

Lifestyle factors that increase risk

One of the biggest breakthroughs of modern medicine has nothing to do with fancy tests or high-tech procedures. It's the discovery that many chronic diseases, including cardiovascular disease, are caused in large part by the way we live. The main lifestyle factors that influence heart disease risk include smoking, being overweight, being sedentary and eating a poor diet.

1 **Smoking** Cigarette smoke delivers hundreds of toxic substances and gases into your lungs and bloodstream. Some of these directly harm the heart. Smoking will cause your arteries to narrow. Carbon monoxide – the same gas your car's exhaust pipe spews out – reduces the amount of oxygen your blood can carry, forcing your heart to work harder than normal. It also robs heart muscle of the blood and oxygen it needs to function properly.

Every year in the UK, more than 114,000 people die as a result of smoking – a quarter of them from cardiovascular disease. Smoking increases your risk of atherosclerosis by 50 per cent and speeds up the damage to your arteries by ten years. The earlier you begin smoking and the more you smoke, the greater the danger. Smoke a pack of 20 a day, and your risk of cardiovascular disease is at least twice as high as that of a nonsmoker. Smoke two or more packs, and it climbs to threefold. If you've tried to stop without success, try again. New smoking aids to stopping, such as nicotine patches have been shown to double your odds of succeeding.

So-called secondhand smoke isn't as dangerous as directly inhaled smoke, but it does increase your risk. It is estimated that passive smoking causes 9,700 deaths from cardiovascular disease annually in the UK among people aged over 65.

2 **Being overweight** The nation's weight problem is bad and getting worse. Today, 43 per cent of men and 34 per cent of women are overweight. Another 23 per cent of men and 22 per cent of women are obese, or severely overweight. The number of adults

▼ Key finding

As dangerous as smoking is for men, it may be even more hazardous for women. Smoking lowers the level of oestrogen in a woman's body – a worry, since many experts believe oestrogen protects women from cardiovascular disease before menopause. Women who smoke and use oral contraceptives, especially women over the age of 35, have higher rates of heart disease than nonsmokers. Although no one knows exactly why, smoking in combination with using oral contraceptives seems to increase blood pressure and cholesterol levels.

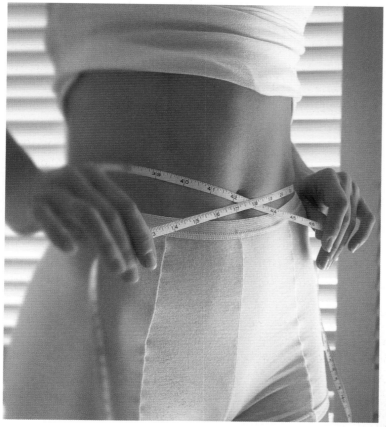

Losing just 4 per cent of your body weight can significantly lower your total cholesterol.

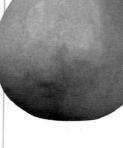

who are obese has doubled in less than 10 years. People in the UK are among the most overweight and obese in the world. All that excess weight adds to heart disease risk because even body fat needs oxygen and nutrients, which are supplied by blood. More fat requires more blood, which leads to high blood pressure. Being overweight also increases the possibility of diabetes. And the simple fact that your body is forced to carry more weight than it was built for strains your heart, adding to the risk of congestive heart failure in people with cardiovascular disease.

3 Being sedentary Being sedentary increases the risk of diabetes and high blood pressure. Couch potatoes are also more likely to be overweight. And when people aren't active, their heart muscles get out of shape, just like the rest of their muscles. That can make the heart more vulnerable to damage.

Studies show that being sedentary doubles your risk of suffering a heart attack. Yet more than seven out of ten of us don't get the recommended dose of exercise (at least 30 minutes of activities like

FAST FACT

Are you shaped more like an apple or a pear? If your body fat is distributed mostly around your stomach (instead of your buttocks, hips, and thighs), you're at greater risk of heart disease.

brisk walking most days of the week). Four out of five women report doing no physical activity. If you spend most of your time sitting, at work or at home, it's high time to get your heart pumping.

Deadly combinations

It's obvious that the more risk factors you have, the greater your odds of developing heart disease or, if you already have it, of suffering a heart attack or stroke. But some factors, when added together, create a combined risk that's greater than you'd expect. Having high cholesterol and smoking, for example, seems to be a particularly menacing combination. High cholesterol is particularly dangerous for people who have diabetes or who are obese. It is also a cause of strokes. Although people in the UK are becoming more aware of the dangers of smoking and being overweight, a survey by Cholesterol UK, a joint initiative by the charities Heart UK and the British Cardiac Patients' Association, reveals that many people are still confused about the danger of high cholesterol levels and do not recognize that raised levels are a major risk factor.

Luckily, there's a bright side. By getting rid of just one risk factor – such as smoking – you will take some of the sting out of other dangers, such as high cholesterol. Eliminate two risk factors and you may gain more than double the benefits for your efforts.

> Most people affected by coronary heart disease have more than one risk factor.

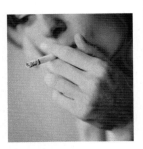

Beating the big three

In the years since researchers identified high blood pressure, high cholesterol and smoking as the principal enemies of the heart, we've made big strides in getting them under control.

But plenty of people remain at risk. Cholesterol UK recently warned that, for instance, two out of three adults over the age of 45 have unhealthy cholesterol levels (but only 5 per cent were aware of the dangers of high cholesterol levels). And some 12 million people in the UK continue to smoke. On top of all this, we're gaining more weight and getting less exercise.

Are we doomed? Certainly not. Making even small inroads against key risk factors, it turns out, can make a big difference.

Consider elevated cholesterol. For every 1 per cent drop in total cholesterol, you get a 2 to 3 per cent reduction in heart disease risk. That's an impressive return on investment. In fact, as long as your level isn't sky-high, there's a good chance you can bring it into the safe zone by making a few lifestyle adjustments.

What's your risk?

By answering a few simple questions, you can get a good idea of your own risk of developing heart disease over the next 10 years. To take this quiz, you'll need to know your blood pressure, total cholesterol and body mass index (see page 131). This test is not for people who have already been diagnosed with cardiovascular disease. Nor does it take the place of a medical examination and doctor's advice. To calculate your risk, add the numbers beside the boxes you've checked.

I am
- Male under 40 1
- Male 40 or older. 2
- Female and have not gone through menopause 1
- Female and have gone through menopause 2

My BMI is
- 19 to 24. 0
- 25 to 29. 1
- 30 or higher 2

I exercise
- More than 30 minutes most days of the week 0
- Up to 30 minutes most days of the week 1
- Very little 2

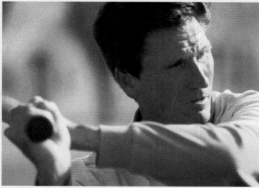

My total cholesterol is
- 3mmol/l or below 0
- 4mmol/l to 5mmol/l 1
- Above 5mmol/l 2

My blood pressure is
- Below 120/80. 0
- Between 121/81 and 139/89 1
- Above 140/90. 2

My smoking history is
- Never smoked. 0
- Quit more than three years ago 1
- Don't smoke but live with people who do 2
- Quit less than three years ago. 2
- Currently smoke 3

I have high blood sugar levels or diabetes
- No 0
- Yes 2

My family history is
- No known family history of early heart attacks 0
- Mother or sister who had a heart attack before age 65 2
- Father or brother who had a heart attack before age 55 2

A score of **0 to 4** indicates a very low risk of developing heart disease.
A score of **5 to 8** indicates a moderate risk of developing heart disease.
A score of **9 to 17** indicates a high risk of developing heart disease.

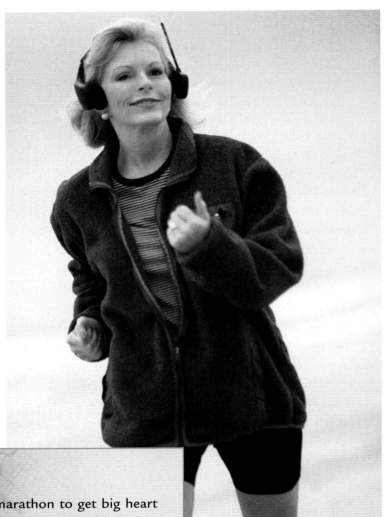

▼ Key finding

You don't have to run a marathon to get big heart benefits. A Harvard University study published in 2001 showed that women who walked just one hour a week lowered their risk of heart disease by 14 per cent. Those who walked for 1½ hours a week reduced their risk by 51 per cent compared with women who rarely walk. Time spent walking, the researchers found, was more important in reducing heart disease risk than the actual walking pace.

What does it take? More sensible eating, is a good way to start. Follow the advice set out by the government's advisory committee on nutrition, which recommends consuming no more than 30 per cent of your calories from fat and only 10 per cent from saturated fats and hydrogenated oils, and if you're like most people, and don't have a genetic predisposition towards high cholesterol levels, you should be able to bring your LDL cholesterol level down by 15 per cent. Adding a few helpings of high-fibre foods can bring the numbers down, too.

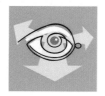

LOOKING AHEAD
New clues to heart disease risk

Although major factors like high blood pressure and elevated cholesterol alert doctors to patients at increased danger of heart disease, they don't identify everyone. Significant numbers of people with no known risk factors have heart attacks. Researchers continue to search for the missing links. So far, several new clues have been identified that may help doctors to pinpoint your risk.

■ **Homocysteine** High blood levels of this amino acid have been linked to increased risk of heart disease. Homocysteine is believed to damage cells that line the coronary arteries. Fortunately folate, a form of B vitamin, keeps levels under control. That's why experts say it's important to get 400 micrograms (mcg) of folate every day. Now that breads and cereals are fortified with the nutrient, most people in the UK get enough in their diets. A daily multivitamin offers added insurance. The belief that folate supplementation may explain the decrease in heart disease that has occurred over the past few decades is controversial and has not been proved.

■ **Lipoprotein (a)** Although low-density lipoproteins, or LDL (the 'bad' cholesterol), are infamous for clogging blood vessels, other lipoproteins may also spell trouble. One currently under investigation, known as Lp(a), has been linked to higher risk of early heart disease. Lp(a) may prevent clots from being dissolved, increasing the danger of a blockage of blood flow to the heart.

■ **Bacteria and viruses** Experts have uncovered evidence that infectious germs may damage blood vessel walls, increasing the risk of arteriosclerosis and blood clots. Culprits include cytomegalovirus, chlamydia and H. pylori. A study published in 2001 looked at 1,018 patients with coronary artery disease. The more germs they tested positive for, the greater their chances of dying from their disease.

■ **C-reactive protein** Inflammation, a natural reaction to injury or infection, may accelerate the process of arteriosclerosis. Scientists have identified a substance called C-reactive protein that serves as a marker for inflammation. In one recent study, men with high levels of the protein had a three times higher risk of heart attack. Some cardiologists now test for C-reactive protein in patients with cardiovascular disease, although others question the value of the results.

■ **HPA-2 Met** A common gene variation dubbed HPA-2 Met makes blood stickier and more likely to clot, according to a 2001 study by scientists in Finland. Men with this trait were found to have double the risk of sudden cardiac death. The gene may also predispose men to coronary thrombosis, or a blood clot in the heart. There is currently no screening test for HPA-2 Met. If anyone in your family has died of premature cardiac arrest, it's important to be screened for other known risk factors, such as high blood pressure and elevated cholesterol. Eventually, researchers believe that genetic tests will play a key role in identifying people at increased risk of heart disease.

A Canadian study showed that a diet that gets more than one-third of its calories from fruit, vegetables, and nuts can lower LDL cholesterol by a remarkable 33 per cent.

The next step is to get moving, and you'll coax those numbers down even farther. When volunteers in a recent Stanford University study switched to a low-fat diet, their LDL levels fell by 7 to 11 per cent. When they added exercise – walking or jogging ten miles a week – the numbers tumbled almost twice as far.

The most important benefit of exercise is its ability to boost HDL, the 'good' cholesterol. In another Stanford study, volunteers who walked or jogged nine miles a week saw their HDL levels climb 13 per cent.

Add it all up, and research shows that with lifestyle changes alone, most individuals can bring elevated cholesterol levels down by 20 to 30 per cent.

Hot topic: Syndrome X: The Feared Foursome

Experts have long known that the more risk factors a person has, the greater the danger of heart disease. But Dr Gerald Reaven, a researcher at Stanford University School of Medicine, believes that one distinct quartet of factors may be especially dangerous.

The combination includes high blood pressure, high triglycerides, low HDL (the so-called 'good' cholesterol) and obesity. Together, these four factors, dubbed metabolic syndrome, or Syndrome X, dramatically increase a person's chances of developing coronary artery disease.

At the core of Syndrome X is insulin resistance, a condition in which cells don't respond to insulin normally. To compensate, the body churns out extra insulin in order to bring the amount of blood sugar, or glucose, in the bloodstream under control by moving it into cells.

This extra insulin may in turn damage the interior lining of blood vessels, increasing the threat of heart attack.

According to the long-running Quebec Cardiovascular Study, every 30 per cent increase in insulin is associated with a 70 per cent increase in the risk of heart disease over a period of five years.

If you have the four risk factors that make up the syndrome, it may be particularly important for your doctor to monitor your blood glucose levels, cholesterol levels and blood pressure. Weight loss and exercise are especially important.

For people with insulin resistance, Dr Reaven advises against a low-fat, high-carbohydrate diet, since people with insulin resistance have to secrete more insulin in order to process carbohydrates. High-protein diets also increase insulin secretion. But dietary fat has no effect on insulin levels. Therefore, Dr. Reaven advises a relatively high-fat diet made up of 40 per cent fats (30 to 35 per cent being unsaturated fats that are healthy for your heart), 45 per cent carbohydrates and 15 per cent protein.

That's enough to keep many people with high cholesterol from needing cholesterol-lowering drugs. Even for those who do need medication, getting heart smart can help to reduce the dose.

Will it work for you?

Diet and exercise efforts don't have the same effect on everyone. Some people can make a small change and see a big result. Others can work hard and see only a small improvement. Take cholesterol. Researchers have found that about 20 per cent of adults are 'nonresponders' – that is, their cholesterol levels won't move even on the best diet and exercise regimen. Another 20 per cent, called 'hyper-responders', will never have to worry about their cholesterol levels no matter what they eat.

It may seem unfair, but remember: even if you're among those who can't lower cholesterol levels without medication, a healthier diet and plenty of physical activity have many other health benefits.

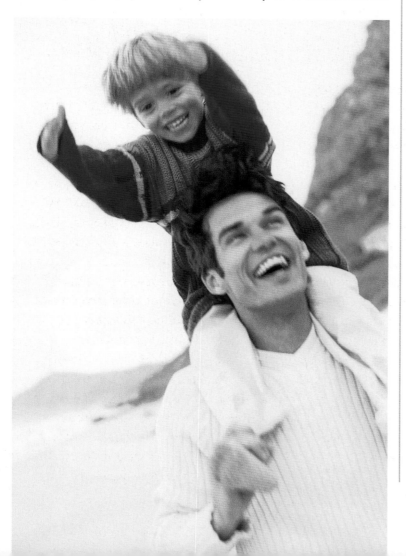

5 THINGS YOU CAN DO TODAY TO LOWER YOUR RISK

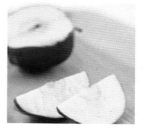

1 Starting today, if you smoke, smoke one less cigarette a day until you're ready to stop.

2 Weigh yourself and work out your BMI (see page 131).

3 Eat one extra piece of fruit and one extra portion of vegetables.

4 Go for a walk. How fast you walk isn't that important. Just try to walk for at least 30 minutes (depending on your current level of fitness).

5 If you don't know your cholesterol level, ask your GP to have it tested.

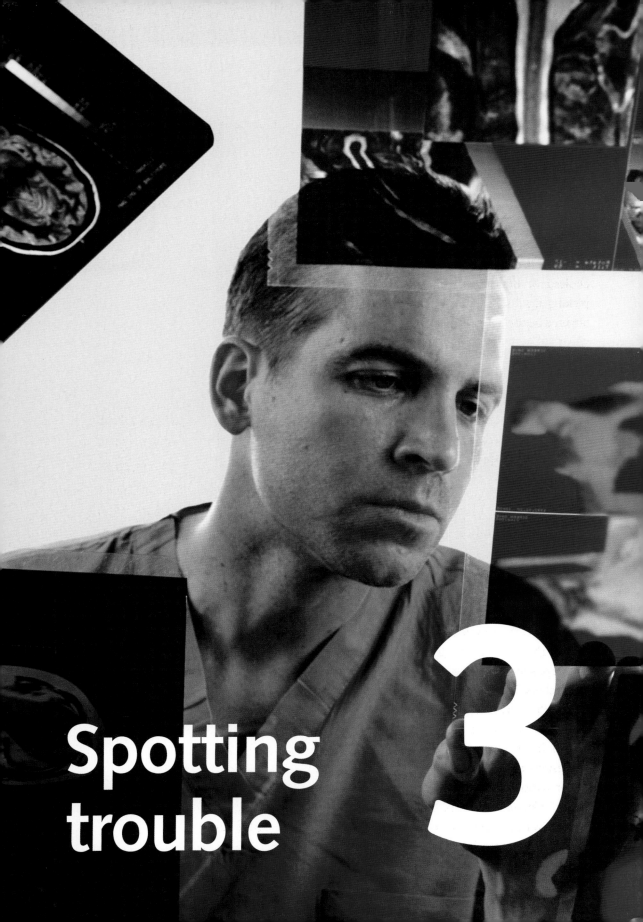

Spotting trouble

3

Too many people don't know they have heart failure until it is too late – a recent study showed that 40 per cent die within a year of diagnosis. Many of those deaths could be prevented. Sophisticated new tests can help your doctor to detect signs of trouble earlier and more accurately than ever.

Using advanced imaging techniques, for instance, physicians can create a detailed map of your heart and arteries, pinpointing cholesterol build-up or damage to heart muscle without ever picking up a scalpel. They can then use this information to take targeted action that could save your life.

Tricky business

Yet, even with the latest advances, diagnosing heart disease can be difficult. One reason is that many different types of heart problem can arise. Some affect the valves of the heart; others interfere with blood flow into the heart; still others may be the result of damage to blood vessels elsewhere in the body.

Complicating matters, more than one problem may occur in the same patient. Someone with atherosclerosis may develop both coronary artery disease (affecting blood flow to the heart) and carotid artery disease (affecting blood flow to the brain). Or a heart attack can lead to congestive heart failure, where damage to the heart interferes with its ability to pump blood efficiently.

Another factor is that coronary artery disease, the leading cause of heart attacks, develops slowly, usually over the course of many years. Atherosclerosis begins when substances such as cholesterol are deposited in fatty streaks on the arteries' inner lining. Researchers have found early signs of this condition in people under 25 – even teenagers. As these fatty deposits accumulate, other substances can adhere to them, including fibrous tissue, various blood components and calcium. These harden into scab-like lesions called plaque, which begin to obstruct blood flow.

For reasons that are only just beginning to be understood, an area of plaque can break loose, plugging up the artery entirely. Alternatively, a blood clot can form on top of plaque, cutting off blood supply to the heart and causing a heart attack.

> Coronary artery disease, the leading cause of heart attacks, develops slowly, usually over the course of many years.

Most people don't know they have a problem until their coronary arteries become so obstructed that blood flow becomes severely restricted. This can cause symptoms such as chest tightness or shortness of breath. Or, if a blood clot abruptly closes off a constricted artery, it can trigger a heart attack.

Early warning signs

The majority of heart attacks don't have to happen. Once coronary artery disease is diagnosed, its progress can be slowed, halted or even reversed through effective treatment and lifestyle changes, such as a healthier diet and more physical activity. An important part of defending your heart is being aware of early symptoms – especially if you know you are at increased risk of heart disease. Not everyone experiences coronary artery disease in the same way, but here are a few common warning signs.

Is it angina?

How do you know if the pain in your chest is angina? It's not always easy even for doctors to recognize angina and distinguish it from other kinds of chest pain. Angina is usually experienced as pressure or squeezing in the middle of the chest behind the breastbone. The pressure, sometimes described as heavy, crushing or like a vice, may radiate up into the throat or jaw or up into the left shoulder and down the left arm. Angina is usually worse in cold weather, during physical activities, following a meal or after emotional stress.

The symptom of chest pressure or shortness of breath can have other causes, of course. Shortness of breath can be triggered

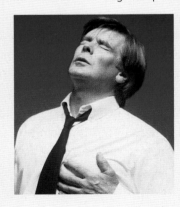

by lung-related illnesses, such as bronchitis or emphysema. Chest pain can be caused by viral infections, strained muscles or even plain old indigestion. Still, symptoms like these shouldn't be taken lightly. If you have them, see your doctor. If he or she believes there is cause for concern, one or more tests may be ordered, such as an electrocardiogram, designed to diagnose specific heart problems.

If you experience chest pain that doesn't subside within a few minutes – especially if you know you are at high risk of coronary artery disease – chew an aspirin and get someone to drive you to an emergency department immediately, or call 999 for an ambulance.

Ischaemia: blood flow reduces to a trickle The first sign of serious trouble from atherosclerosis is ischaemia, which simply means decreased blood flow. 'Myocardial ischaemia' refers to reduced flow of blood through the coronary arteries that feed the heart. Some patients with myocardial ischaemia have symptoms such as a tightness in the chest or weakness when they exert themselves, and these tip off doctors that the heart is beginning to be robbed of oxygen and nutrients.

Angina: a pain in the chest
As the arteries that supply the heart become more and more obstructed, some people experience a form of chest pain called angina. It often occurs first when they are under physical or emotional stress –

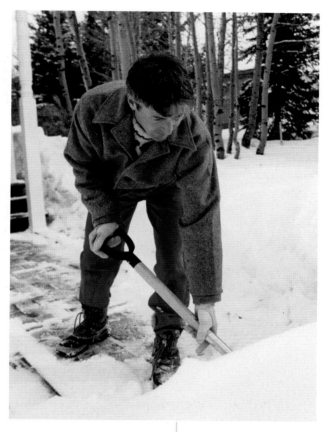

playing squash, for instance, or arguing with a partner. Angina triggered by exercise, sometimes called exertional angina, usually subsides when people stop what they're doing and rest. As the artery blockages become worse, however, angina may happen when people are simply sitting still or even sleeping.

Angina that occurs at rest usually indicates more serious ischaemia. Constricted arteries can no longer supply even the minimal amount of oxygenated blood the heart needs. When angina enters this phase, it is sometimes called unstable angina. The reason is that the blood supply to the heart has become so restricted that a heart attack can occur at almost any time.

Heart attack: when the damage turns deadly

Unfortunately, some patients never experience pain in their chest until the arteries that serve the heart become completely obstructed, cutting off blood flow to parts of the heart and causing a heart attack. This can happen when one of the scab-like plaques breaks free from the artery wall and plugs up a narrowed section of the artery. It can also result when a blood clot forms in an artery

> **Angina** triggered by exercise, sometimes called exertional angina, usually subsides when people stop what they're doing and rest.

already constricted by atherosclerosis. If the blood supply is cut off for long enough – around 30 minutes – heart muscle cells will begin to die.

The British Heart Foundation has identified three common warning signals of a heart attack. They are:

- Uncomfortable pressure, fullness, squeezing or pain in the centre of your chest lasting more than a few minutes. (This feeling of pressure isn't necessarily located right over the heart. It can occur anywhere in the chest.)
- Pain spreading to the shoulders, neck or arms.
- Lightheadedness, fainting, sweating, nausea or shortness of breath, usually accompanied by discomfort in your chest.

Other, less common symptoms include stomach or abdominal pain, difficulty breathing, unexplained anxiety or fatigue and palpitations or cold sweats. Bear in mind that not all of them occur in every heart attack and some come and go.

Unfortunately, of the estimated 270,000 people in the UK who have heart attacks every year, only about 70 per cent get to an emergency department in time. Only 25 per cent telephone for help within an hour of symptoms appearing. If you think you may be having a heart attack, call 999 and then take an aspirin, either chewing it or putting it under your tongue to speed its absorption into the bloodstream, instead of simply swallowing it. Aspirin helps to thin the blood and keep it flowing.

▼ Key finding

Between a third and two-thirds of heart attacks take place away from hospitals and 12,000 people suffer cardiac arrest in public places every year. Many more would survive if more defibrillators were available in public places like airports, shopping centres, stations and office buildings – and if more people were trained in their use. Automatic external defibrillators, or AEDs, are devices used by emergency medical staff to 'shock' the heart of someone in cardiac arrest into beating normally again. Since 2000, the Department of Health has funded the installation of more than 700 AEDs in 110 places in the country, and more are planned. At least 36 lives have been saved as a result.

Heart failure: weak but still beating

A heart attack and heart failure may sound like the same thing, but they represent very different conditions. A heart attack occurs when a blockage in one of the coronary arteries suddenly cuts off blood supply to the heart, causing serious damage to heart muscles. Heart failure, by contrast, typically develops slowly as the heart muscle grows weaker and weaker, becoming less efficient at pumping blood around the

A closer look at lipids

Many university hospitals and major medical centres now offer lipid clinics. These state-of-the-art facilities look beyond standard cholesterol tests at a variety of more subtle clues to heart attack risk.

The reason: standard risk factors account for only about half of all cases of coronary artery disease. Half of all people who develop heart problems, in other words, don't have the usual early warning signs of high blood pressure or elevated cholesterol. At lipid clinics, doctors and researchers use more sophisticated blood tests to try to spot hidden danger signs.

Patients are typically referred to a lipid clinic after being diagnosed with angina or atherosclerosis, after a heart attack or to help them manage diabetes. Experts say it's also a good idea to visit a lipid clinic if you have a strong family history of early heart attacks. One goal of the clinics is to find out why a person with no known risk factors suddenly develops heart disease.

Says Dr Mary Malloy, who heads the lipid clinic at the University of California at San Francisco (UCSF): 'We may see a patient whose total HDL levels look fine, but when we look more closely at the HDL, we discover defects that may get in the way of its transporting cholesterol out of the body.' Researchers may also find defects in LDL particles that prevent them from being cleared from the blood stream normally.

The tests offered at lipid clinics can help doctors to choose the best treatment. Patients who have a certain defect in their LDL may be less sensitive to cholesterol-lowering statin drugs, for instance. In that case, they may fare better on niacin, which improves cholesterol status by raising HDL. Patients who are discovered to have high blood levels of cardiac C-reactive protein, which indicates inflammation, may be treated with an antibiotic. Chronic inflammation can injure the lining of artery walls, making them more susceptible to cholesterol build-up.

Another goal of many lipid clinics is to advance the science of detecting heart disease risk. At UCSF's lipid clinic, researchers are screening blood from 20,000 patients with atherosclerosis to try to find genetic markers associated with increased risk. Already, three genetic disorders have been linked to coronary artery disease.

body. (Despite its name, it does not mean that the heart has stopped working.) The two conditions can be related. Some people who survive a heart attack go on to develop heart failure, for instance. Others may develop heart failure without ever having a heart attack. The most common cause of heart failure is multiple heart attacks. High blood pressure and heart-valve defects can also lead to heart failure. Alcoholism and drug abuse are other causes.

Because the two sides of the heart perform different functions, doctors can often tell which side is failing simply by a patient's symptoms The left side pumps blood that has just been supplied with oxygen from the lungs out into the arteries. If that side isn't working properly, blood and fluid can accumulate in the lungs, causing shortness of breath and persistent coughing. The right chambers of the heart receive blood from the body's tissues. If this side is failing, fluid and pressure build up in the veins that return blood to the heart. The pressure can cause pain in the liver and swelling in the legs. This condition is called congestive heart failure.

Other forms of heart trouble

Coronary artery disease is by far the leading form of heart disease, but there are many other types of cardiovascular problem. Here are four of the most common.

Hot topic: Poor sleepers, beware

Are you a ferocious snorer? Do you wake up feeling exhausted? You may be suffering from sleep apnoea – which could be bad news for your heart. In this condition, breathing stops repeatedly for brief periods during the night. People usually wake up during these lapses, although they may not remember doing so. Scientists have found that sleep apnoea may be associated with increased risk of a variety of cardiovascular diseases, including ischaemia (lack of blood and oxygen to the heart) and heartbeat irregularities.

According to The British Snoring and Sleep Apnoea Association, people with sleep apnoea are much more likely to suffer high blood pressure than those who sleep soundly. It's now thought that nearly 50 per cent of sleep apnoea patients have hypertension. Those with the most severe sleep apnoea seem to have the highest blood

pressure – and often the most difficulty in controlling it. Snoring alone doesn't seem to pose a problem. But if snoring occurs along with sleep apnoea – and obesity – the risk of high blood pressure increases.

Why sleep disorders are linked to heart disease is still something of a mystery. But treating sleep apnoea by opening up the airways (usually by wearing a special mask that delivers pressurized air, or through surgery) can bring blood pressure down. If you often wake during the night and feel sleepy during the day, mention your symptoms to your doctor.

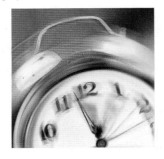

Congenital heart disease Every year in the UK, about 5,000 babies are born with a heart condition – that's about one in every 145 babies. They have what is called a congenital heart defect. Congenital defects are more common in children of mothers with congenital heart problems. Often the causes are unknown, although infections during pregnancy, or the mother's use of drugs or alcohol, can damage the heart.Problems can include malformed heart valves, abnormalities that impede the flow of blood through vessels, and defects in the structure of the heart. Congenital heart defects can be diagnosed in the uterus as early as the 16th week of life. Once a baby is born, surgeons are often able to correct the defect. Between five and seven children in every 1,000 develop the disease after birth.

Cardiomyopathy Poor nutrition, inflammation caused by viral infections, pregnancy complications and other factors can cause damage to the heart muscle, called cardiomyopathy. This in turn can reduce the heart's pumping efficiency. In 80 per cent of cases, physicians cannot identify a cause. When the cause is unknown, researchers call the condition idiopathic. Unlike most other forms of heart disease, cardiomyopathy can affect young people. It is the cause of 200 to 400 deaths a year – about eight people a week – and is one of the leading causes of sudden cardiac arrest.

Heartbeat irregularities Almost everyone's heart skips a beat now and then or produces a double beat in the place of a single beat. Most of the time these minor irregularities, called arrhythmia, don't signal trouble. But certain types of arrhythmia caused by coronary artery disease can pose a serious threat. In ventricular fibrillation, for instance, the ventricles (lower chambers of the heart) rapidly contract in an uncoordinated way, causing the heart to stop pumping. Around 700,000 people in the UK suffer from arrhythmia. Medications or pacemakers can control many forms of arrhythmia.

Diseases of the heart valves Four valves control the flow of blood into and out of the heart. Blood entering the heart flows through the tricuspid valve into the right ventricle and, from there, through the pulmonary valve to the lungs, where it picks up oxygen. Returning from the lungs, newly oxygenated blood enters the left atrium and passes through the mitral valve to the left ventricle. It's then pumped through the aortic valve and out into the body. Congenital defects, infections or the build-up of calcium can interfere with the function of heart valves, making the heart less efficient. Most valve problems can be treated with drugs or repaired with surgery, including the insertion of mechanical valves.

FAST FACT
In a small study by Oxford University, it was found that 50 per cent of men and 58 per cent of women die within 28 days of having had a heart attack.

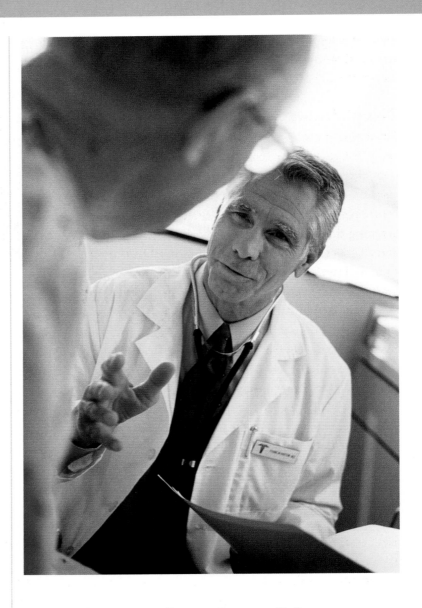

Assessing your heart's condition

The answers to a few simple questions and results of tests done right in your doctor's surgery can provide a surprisingly detailed picture of the state of your heart and your overall health. During the examination, the doctor or cardiologist will talk with you about how you're feeling, your family history and any risk factors you may have. He or she will also want to know what kinds of symptoms you're having. It's essential to answer the questions as completely and honestly as you can and to mention any concerns you have. After all, a symptom you've been experiencing may provide your doctor with a vital clue.

That's why it's a good idea to make a list of the things you want to cover and bring it with you, so that you don't forget something that may be important.

The physical examination

The goal of a physical examination is to learn as much about what's going on inside the body as possible from the outside. Just looking at skin colour, for instance, can tell a doctor whether the heart is delivering enough oxygen to the tissues in the body. Listening through a stethoscope can indicate how the four chambers of the heart are working together. During a physical test, your doctor will check the health of your heart and blood vessels using five standard tests.

I **Blood pressure**. This familiar test uses a cuff wrapped around your upper arm and inflated to create pressure. The cuff is attached to a gauge filled with mercury. By listening to your pulse when the cuff is inflated and as it is deflated, your doctor notes when a heartbeat can no longer be heard and then when it becomes audible again. The mercury level (or on newer digital types, a gauge or dial) indicates pressure when your heart beats and when it rests.

2 **Heart rate and rhythm** By feeling your pulse with his or her fingertips, your doctor can spot signs of an irregular heart rhythm. He or she can also determine your resting heart rate, or the number of times your heart beats each minute.

3 **Venous pulses** A doctor can actually see your pulse by looking at a vein on your neck called the jugular. By observing how this vein expands as your heart beats, your doctor can estimate the pressure on the right side of your heart and spot signs that there may be extra fluid in your cardiovascular system.

4 **Oedema** Excess fluid may accumulate in your legs if your heart isn't pumping effectively. This, called oedema, can cause visible swelling

LOOKING AHEAD

Before you have angioplasty

A new test to measure the pressure of blood flow through clogged arteries could help doctors identify patients who would benefit most from treatment. The experimental technique uses a catheter to measure blood flow at the same time as an angiogram (see page 54) is performed. Studies have shown that if blood flow is only minimally reduced – even in patients with atherosclerosis – opening up the artery with balloon angioplasty offers no benefit.

If blood flow is moderately reduced, however – even if the blockage itself doesn't appear to be substantial – angioplasty can be life-saving.

TERMS TO KNOW

ANGINA Chest pain caused by blockage of the arteries that supply blood to the heart

ANGIOGRAM An X-ray test that uses dye injected into blood vessels to create an image of the coronary arteries

ARRHYTHMIA Abnormal heart rhythm

CARDIAC ENZYMES Substances in the heart that can provide a signal when heart muscle is damaged

CARDIOMYOPATHY Any structural or functional disease of the heart muscle

DEFIBRILLATOR A device that delivers an electrical charge designed to 'shock' an arrested heart into beating again

ECHOCARDIOGRAM Non-invasive test that uses ultrasound waves to create an image of the heart

ELECTROCARDIOGRAM (ECG) A diagnostic test using electrodes to record the heart's electrical activity

HEART FAILURE A condition in which the heart can no longer pump blood adequately

MYOCARDIAL ISCHAEMIA Caused when too little blood and oxygen reach the heart muscle as a result of blockage to the arteries

OEDEMA Swelling caused by the accumulation of fluid, which can be a symptom of heart failure

PLAQUE A deposit of fat and other substances in the inner lining of an artery wall

RADIOISOTOPE SCANNING A diagnostic test (also called radionuclide scanning) that uses radioactive dye injected into the bloodstream to create a detailed picture of the heart and arteries

SILENT ISCHAEMIA A blockage of blood flow that causes no symptoms

SPHYGMOMANOMETER An instrument used to measure blood pressure

STRESS TEST An electrocardiogram conducted while the patient is walking and/or running on a treadmill

around your ankles, shins, thighs, lower back, abdomen or hands. To test for fluid retention, your doctor presses on the skin to see how far it goes in, creating an indentation.

5 Heartbeat, breathing and blood flow Placing a stethoscope on the skin above your heart, your doctor can gauge how well your heart valves are opening and closing. Telltale sounds provide information about possible heart defects.

By listening to your chest through the stethoscope while you breathe in and out, your doctor is alert to sounds that may indicate that extra fluid has accumulated in your lungs.

Placing the stethoscope over other parts of your body, he or she can hear the sound of blood flowing in major vessels. A whispering sound, usually called a bruit, is a sign of abnormal turbulence in blood flow.

Diagnostic tests

When doctors find signs of trouble during a physical exam, they turn to more sophisticated tests to learn the precise cause, including blood tests and procedures used to create images of the heart and blood vessels.

Secrets from the blood

Human blood reveals an astonishing amount of information about the body, from the state of the immune system to the functioning of organs such as the liver and kidneys. A simple blood test can reveal your total cholesterol level as well as HDL and LDL cholesterol – an important gauge of the health of your blood vessels. Blood tests can also uncover other risk factors, such as abnormal homocysteine levels and the presence of enzymes that signal high levels of inflammation.

If your doctor suspects your heart may have suffered damage as a result of artery blockages, blood tests can indicate the extent of injury. Blood levels of certain heart enzymes rise in the hours following damage to heart muscle. Four cardiac enzymes your doctor may test for are creatine kinase, lactate dehydrogenase, troponin-I and troponin-T.

Electrocardiograms

The test most commonly used to diagnose heart conditions is the electrocardiogram, which is often abbreviated to ECG. Electrocardiograms can be performed in three basic ways: a resting ECG; an exercise ECG; and an ambulatory, or walking, ECG.

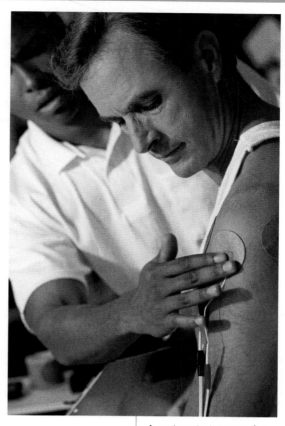

In a stress test, or exercise ECG, a faster heart rate makes it easier to detect ischaemia (reduced blood and oxygen supply to the heart) and rhythm abnormalities brought on by exercise.

I Resting ECG If your doctor suspects that you are suffering from heart disease, the first test is likely to be a resting ECG, which creates a graph or tracing of your heart's electrical signals while you remain still.

WHAT TO EXPECT First, electrodes are placed at various locations on your body, usually the ankles, wrists and chest. They are often covered with a sticky gel that ensures good contact. Wires from the electrodes transmit electrical signals to a small device that makes a tracing of your heart rate and rhythm. The test usually takes about 5 minutes.

WHAT THE RESULTS SHOW ECGs help doctors to diagnose irregular heart rhythms, damage from a heart attack or any other heart abnormalities. ECGs can also indicate signs of inadequate blood and oxygen supply to specific regions of heart muscle.

2 Exercise ECG In some cases, signs and symptoms of heart problems show up during exertion. If the resting ECG fails to show any abnormalities, your doctor may prescribe an exercise ECG, more commonly known as a stress test.

WHAT TO EXPECT Electrodes are attached just as they are for a resting ECG. You'll be asked to walk and then perhaps run on a treadmill to raise your heart rate. The treadmill starts slowly. Gradually the pace and the incline are increased in order to put more demand on your heart. Don't worry: you will be monitored constantly during the test. The moment you feel pain or become tired or too short of breath to continue, the test will be stopped. An exercise ECG, which is usually done in a clinic or hospital, takes about half an hour.

WHAT THE RESULTS SHOW Like a resting ECG, the exercise treadmill test can turn up a variety of abnormalities in heart rhythm. If you experience chest pressure or pain while on the treadmill, the test confirms that you have angina. Your doctor can gauge how severe the angina is, based on how long you remain on the treadmill before the pain occurs.

3 Ambulatory ECG If you suffer from intermittent heartbeat abnormalities, your doctor may recommend an ambulatory ECG, also sometimes called a Holter monitor. This test records heart activity over a 24-hour period.

WHAT TO EXPECT Electrodes are connected to a recording device about the size of a paperback book, which you'll be asked to wear over 24 hours, even while you sleep. As you go about your every-day business, the device records your heart's electrical patterns. Your doctor may also ask you to keep a diary of what you're doing and any symptoms you experience.

Later, the data, will be analysed, correlating your heartbeat patterns to what you were doing and how you felt.

WHAT THE RESULTS SHOW By providing continuous monitoring of the heart, an ambulatory ECG enables doctors to see abnormalities

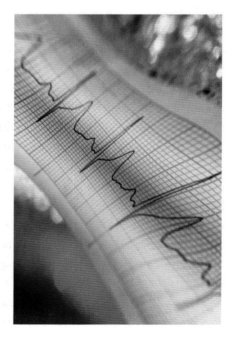

An ECG trace shows the electrical activity of the heart as the upper chamber contracts, then the lower. In between beats, the heart rests.

that may occur only once in a while, in a 24-hour period. It also allows them to see how specific activities affect your heart, providing important clues about which ones trigger abnormal heart rhythms, for instance.

Electrophysiologic tests

Like an ECG, an electrophysiologic test uses electrodes to measure electrical signals emanating from the heart. Instead of being placed on the skin, the electrodes are inserted through veins and, sometimes, through arteries directly into the heart's chambers to record electrical signals from within the heart.

It is a more invasive procedure. In order to gauge whether a particular drug or surgical repair will help to stop the disturbance, cardiologists some-times trigger abnormal heart rhythms intentionally Electrophysiologic tests are sometimes used when ECG results are inconclusive.

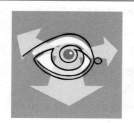

LOOKING AHEAD

The closest look yet inside arteries

A new form of high-resolution magnetic resonance imaging (MRI), called 'black blood MRI', recently created the most detailed images ever recorded of the inside of coronary arteries in living patients. The technology can be used to pinpoint potential trouble spots in arteries long before symptoms of athero-sclerosis show up, say researchers at Mount Sinai School of Medicine in New York. Experts hope the technique will allow doctors to identify vulnerable artery plaques before they rupture. They could then more precisely target treatments to prevent heart attacks. Though promising, the test remains experimental.

WHAT TO EXPECT The test is usually performed in a special surgery or laboratory. The area where the electrode catheters will be inserted (usually the groin) is scrubbed and shaved. Typically, three or four catheters – each one about as thick as a strand of spaghetti – are inserted at the same time. If your doctor uses a small electrical charge to trigger an arrhythmia, you may feel an unusual heartbeat or a fluttering feeling in your heart. When the test begins, the table you are lying on will be horizontal. During the test, it may be tilted to an upright position so that your heart's response to changes in position can be assessed. The process can take anywhere from an hour to more than 4 hours.

WHAT THE RESULTS SHOW Electrophysiologic studies produce a map of the heart's electrical system, showing how nerve impulses are conducted from one part of the heart to another. They help doctors to determine where, along the conduction system, the electrical impulses that produce your heartbeat are going awry and which treatments can be used to fix the problem.

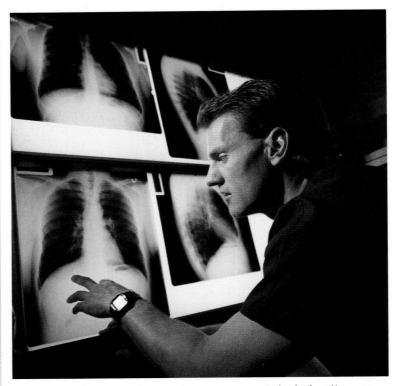

A simple chest X-ray can reveal calcium deposits, heart enlargement and lung changes caused by heart failure.

Imaging techniques

Doctors have at their disposal a variety of tools for creating images of the heart and circulatory system, from simple X-rays to highly sophisticated tests that provide three-dimensional and even moving pictures of the heart. The imaging tests your doctor is most likely to recommend include:

| Chest X-ray A chest X-ray, just like the kind used to see the condition of your lungs, can provide important clues to the state of your heart.

WHAT TO EXPECT After removing clothes and jewellery above your waist, you'll stand against a plate that contains X-ray film. X-rays will be aimed at your chest. They will penetrate different tissues in different ways, creating an image of bone, heart muscle, and the outline of your lungs on X-ray film.

WHAT THE RESULTS SHOW X-rays provide a picture of the size and shape of your heart. They can also reveal calcium

TROUBLESHOOTING TIP

Diagnostic tests don't have to be frightening.

■ **If you have questions about why a test is being done, ask your doctor.**

■ **If you're worried about what a test will be like, ask for a description of exactly what will be done and how it will feel.**

■ **If you feel very anxious about a test, say so. Your doctor may be able to give you medication to help you to calm down.**

deposits that may indicate heart disease or injury, as well as provide information about the health of your lungs.

2 Radioisotope scanning Like X-rays, radioisotope scans use very low levels of radiation to create images of the heart. But while an X-ray creates a picture by passing radiation through the body from an outside source, a radioisotope scan uses radioactive material injected into the bloodstream. Special cameras detect the material as it passes through the heart and arteries, providing vital information about coronary blood flow.

Diagnosing a stroke

A stroke occurs when the blood supply to parts of the brain is interrupted. There are two main types of stroke. In an ischaemic stroke, blood flow is blocked as a result of atherosclerosis, sometimes compounded by a blood clot. Haemorrhagic strokes occur when a blood vessel in the brain ruptures. A variety of tests allow doctors to zero in on the area of the brain that was affected and assess the kind of damage that occurred.

■ Taking pictures

Several of the same tests that help doctors to diagnose heart disease can detect strokes. CT scans, for instance, are used to determine the kind of stroke and where it has occurred. MRIs create highly detailed images of the brain, pinpointing the location and size of the affected area. Angiograms, very similar to those used to create an image of the coronary arteries, can also be used to make detailed maps of blood flow in the brain, showing which areas have been robbed of their blood supply.

■ Tracing electrical activity

Doctors can also trace the brain's electrical activity with an electroencephalogram, or EEG. Electrodes placed at strategic locations on the scalp detect electrical impulses in various parts of the brain. By recording the intensity, duration, frequency and location of electrical activity, EEGs help doctors to assess damage.

■ Listening in

Tests that measure sound waves also provide important clues. A device that emits ultrasound, for instance, can be used to record the speed of blood cells flowing through the carotid arteries, the two main vessels that supply blood to the brain. In another test, called a carotid phonoangiogram, doctors place a small microphone against the neck to record the sound of blood flowing through these arteries. The microphone is sensitive enough to pick up the difference between normal blood flow and the sound of turbulence that may indicate a blockage.

WHAT TO EXPECT Although the injection of radioactive material sounds a little worrying, it's very safe. The amount of radiation is roughly what you receive during a standard chest X-ray. The material, called a tracer, is injected into your arm. The test may be done while you are resting, or you may be asked to exercise on a treadmill or stationary bike before the tracer material is injected. Afterwards you'll lie still while a camera takes a series of pictures from different angles, which can last up to 25 minutes. This type of test is more accurate than an exercise ECG and is sometimes used when the results of an ECG are inconclusive or when more information is needed. It is also considerably more expensive.

WHAT THE RESULTS SHOW The detailed images of your heart and the blood vessels that supply it can reveal the extent of damage to heart muscles after a heart attack or measure the amount of blood that passes through the heart each time it beats. A form of radioisotope scanning called single photon emission computed tomography (SPECT) can be used to create a three-dimensional functional image of the heart. These scans are extremely accurate in detecting ischaemias, or areas of restricted blood flow.

3 Coronary angiography Angiography involves the injection of a special dye into the arteries that supply the heart, allowing the heart's activity to be recorded by X-ray cameras. This is the most common test used to diagnose coronary artery disease. Angiography can reveal blockages or narrowed areas that aren't visible on normal X-rays.

WHAT TO EXPECT A local anaesthetic is used to numb the area, then a narrow tube called a catheter is inserted into an artery in the groin – or it may be inserted at the wrist or elbow. The catheter is fed through the artery until it reaches a coronary artery. Dye is injected, and a series of X-rays is taken. The insertion of

Coronary angiography reveals a section of an artery (encircled) that has been narrowed by coronary artery disease.

the catheter is usually painless. Some patients experience a few palpitations when the tube reaches the heart. The test, which takes about 40 minutes, is usually done at an outpatient clinic. The injection site may be bruised and tender for a few days.

WHAT THE RESULTS SHOW An angiogram of the heart provides a detailed image of the condition of the vessels that supply blood to the heart, including any blockages. Angiography is typically used when doctors believe a patient may benefit from heart surgery or angioplasty, a technique that opens blocked vessels.

4 Echocardiography This procedure can offer a non-invasive way to look at your heart. Instead of X-rays and dyes, echocardiography uses echoes. Sound waves, called ultrasound, are directed at the heart via a microphone-like device known as a transducer. By detecting the echoes that bounce back from the heart, it is possible to trace a picture of your heart while it is beating.

WHAT TO EXPECT An echocardiogram is usually carried out at a hospital. The technician or doctor will apply gel or oil to your chest to improve the transmission of ultrasound waves. The test is usually painless, although sometimes the transducer must be held very firmly against the skin, which can feel a bit uncomfortable. Echocardiography typically takes about 15 minutes to an hour.

WHAT THE RESULTS SHOW The images produced by an echocardiogram can reveal damage to the heart muscle, abnormal blood flow, valve problems and other conditions.

▼ Key finding

Research shows that ultrafast MRI, a new form of high-resolution magnetic resonance imaging, can detect most diseased coronary arteries, might possibly spare patients from undergoing an angiogram, which is a much more invasive test. MRI has been used to examine very large blood vessels for years. But only recently has it been adapted to produce images of the relatively small coronary arteries. According to a study published in the December 2001 issue of *The New England Journal of Medicine*, ultrafast MRI detected every diseased coronary artery in 75 per cent of patients studied. It ruled out coronary artery disease accurately between 81 per cent and 100 per cent of the time.

Advanced imaging techniques

Several tests can create even more detailed images of the heart, including three-dimensional pictures. These include computed tomography (CT), magnetic resonance imaging (MRI) and positron emission tomography (PET). New advances are making them more accurate than ever. CT scans use X-rays, but instead of taking a single picture, the X-ray machine is rotated rapidly around the body so that images are captured from all angles. This allows doctors to view internal organs in cross-section. An even newer test called cine-computed tomography creates a three-dimensional moving image of the heart. MRIs can record small energy signals that are emitted by the atoms that make up cells in different body tissues. PET scans, the newest diagnostic tool, and one that is currently used mostly for research purposes, detect emissions from subatomic particles. They can determine how well portions of the heart muscle are functioning after a heart attack, helping doctors to decide whether or not to repair a blockage of an artery supplying blood to that area.

WHAT TO EXPECT You'll lie flat on a movable table. In a CT scan, the table is passed slowly through a giant ring that scans your body from all angles. In an MRI scan, the table is moved through a stationary chamber. You will be required to lie very still while inside the magnetic chamber. The operation of the magnet is very noisy. The procedure, which is painless, can take half an hour or more. In a PET scan, a small amount of radioactive material is injected into the blood before the scan, which takes about an hour.

WHAT THE RESULTS SHOW High-tech scans can be used to evaluate ischaemia and look at diseases of the heart valves.

An ounce of prevention

The diagnostic tests available now provide an astonishingly clear portrait of the state of the heart and circulatory system, helping doctors to pinpoint the source of trouble so that they can treat it more effectively. That's excellent news, of course. But researchers also hope that they can encourage people to prevent cardiovascular problems from developing in the first place. One of the best ways to do that is to stop smoking – see the next chapter.

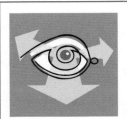

LOOKING AHEAD

Early warning sign of heart attack

Researchers may soon be able to identify plaques on arteries that are vulnerable to rupturing and blocking blood flow, possibly triggering a heart attack. In 2001, researchers at Germany's Bonn University injected into the bloodstream magnetic molecules that bind to fibrin, a substance that forms in plaques. MRI scans were then used to see where the molecules had accumulated. The technique may one day help doctors to determine the degree of danger and to decide how to treat patients with vulnerable plaques.

REAL PEOPLE, REAL WISDOM

A doctor's story

The signs of trouble were there, Dr Stephen Weiss realizes, if only he'd been paying enough attention to notice them. 'I realize now that for almost two years I'd been experiencing what doctors call exertional angina – chest pain that comes on during physical exertion,' 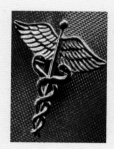 says Dr Weiss, 46, a general practitioner in northern California. 'My chest would feel tight, and I'd be short of breath after climbing hills on my bicycle. But frankly, I figured I was just getting older.'

Then after a bout of flu, Dr. Weiss noticed he was having much more than the usual trouble getting back into shape. He would experience pain and tightness in his chest just walking to another department during work.

It wasn't until a few days later, at home, that he realized something was seriously wrong. 'I'd gone out to get a package, and by the time I got back inside I was so weak I had to lie down on the floor.' His wife insisted he go to the emergency department, where he was examined by a cardiologist. 'At first glance everything looked normal. My blood pressure. My pulse rate. The chest X-ray. My cardiac C-reactive enzymes. My cholesterol levels.'

The cardiologist conducted a stress test, or treadmill electrocardiogram. Three months earlier, Dr Weiss had completed a 3-hour bike ride with no trouble. Now he could barely last for 10 minutes on the treadmill. The cardiologist ordered an angiogram, a test that uses injected dye to create a detailed image of the arteries that supply the heart. When Dr Weiss saw the results, he knew he was lucky to be alive. One of his coronary arteries was almost 99 per cent blocked. At any time, a blood clot could have closed it off completely, triggering a heart attack.

Finally the cardiologist did an angioplasty, which uses a small inflated balloon to widen the blocked vessel. Then a metal device called a stent was inserted to help to prevent the artery from closing up again.

Six months later, Dr Weiss is working full-time again and beginning to return to his normal activity level. But things aren't the same. For starters, he and his family have dramatically changed the way they eat, adopting a low-fat diet with much more fruit, vegetables and whole-grain foods. The goal: to limit the damage his coronary artery disease had caused by following a strict diet and getting back to exercise. He's also become serious about controlling stress by finding time for himself and using relaxation techniques like meditation on a regular basis.

'It's been scary,' he admits. 'But it's also made me a different and, I hope, a better doctor. I find myself spending a little more time with my patients, listening more closely to what they're telling me. I missed the first signs that something was wrong with me. I don't want to miss them in my patients.'

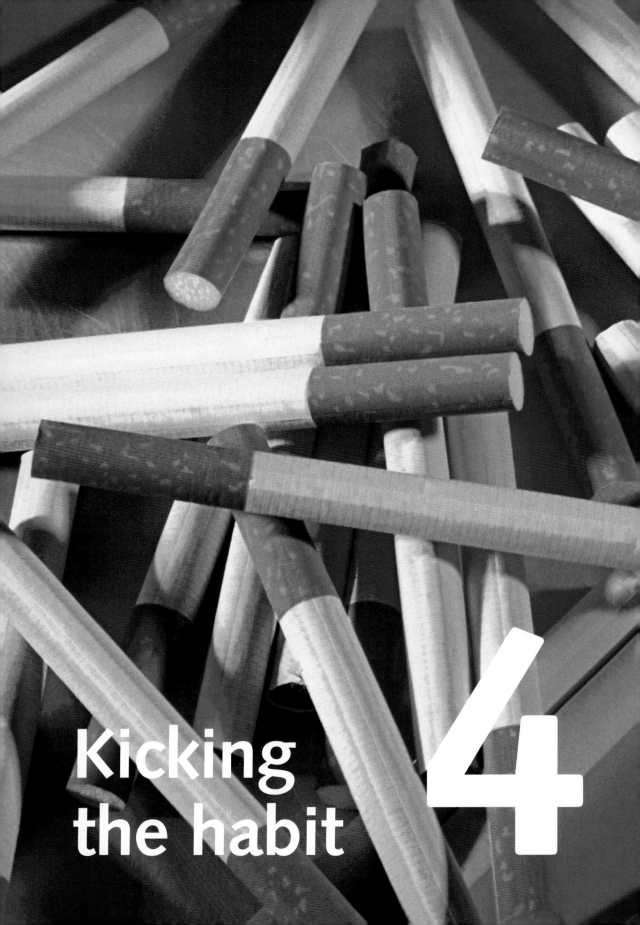

Kicking the habit

4

Smoking is especially bad for your heart. It causes arteries to narrow, just as high blood pressure does. It wreaks havoc with the ratio of 'good' cholesterol to 'bad' cholesterol in your blood and puts you at higher risk of the blood clots that cause heart attacks and strokes. The good news is that even if you're a long-term smoker, you can substantially cut your risk of premature death by stopping today.

You have probably promised yourself that you will stop – in fact, at any given moment, four out of five smokers say they want to do just that. But breaking free of a tobacco addiction is anything but easy. On the other hand, 12 million ex-smokers in the UK prove that it can be done.

If you've tried and failed to quit, take heart: most people attempt to give up smoking two or three times before they succeed for good. Those early efforts aren't failures; they're more like dress rehearsals – a chance to discover which strategies work for you. And quitting today is easier than ever before thanks to a variety of products aimed at curing your nicotine addiction, from nicotine patches and gum to medication that takes the edge off your cravings.

The benefits of quitting are huge, and you'll start enjoying some right away. Food tastes better. Your mouth feels fresher. You'll begin to have more energy. More important, after a year of being smoke-free, your risk of heart disease will fall by half. Three to four years after you stop, you'll be at no greater risk than someone who has never smoked, according to ASH (Action on Smoking and Health).

> Three to four years after you stop, you'll be at no greater risk of heart disease than someone who has never smoked.

Hard habit to break

Why are cigarettes so difficult to give up? First, nicotine is addictive. For some people it can be as addictive as heroin or cocaine, according to the Royal College of Physicians. Smokers who try to quit may feel irritable, light-headed and anxious. Many have trouble concentrating for the first week or two.

Second, smoking becomes tied to one's daily routines, creating a psychological dependence. Lighting up may be part of the morning ritual, for instance. Many smokers associate smoking with meals and find themselves craving a cigarette after lunch or dinner. Others can't resist a cigarette when they're out drinking with friends. These obstacles can also be overcome. By changing your routines and avoiding situations you associate with smoking, you can steer clear of psychological triggers.

FAST FACT
Twenty per cent of all coronary artery disease in the UK is blamed on smoking.

A weighty matter

One reason some people hesitate to quit is a fear of weight gain. Not everyone who gives up smoking puts on weight but, on average, smokers who do stop put on 7–14lb during the first six months. Scientists don't fully understand why. One explanation may simply be that food tastes better, so your appetite increases. Another may be that smoking speeds up your metabolism, which causes the body to burn extra calories. When you quit, your metabolism slows down just a bit.

All else being equal, scientists estimate that the average person burns about 200 more calories a day when smoking than when not. How can you make up the difference? One brisk 30-minute walk will do the trick. Or make a determined effort to resist a single high-calorie snack, such as a chocolate bar. Finally, remember that it's far better to carry a few extra pounds than to poison your body with tobacco and suffer all the attendant harms.

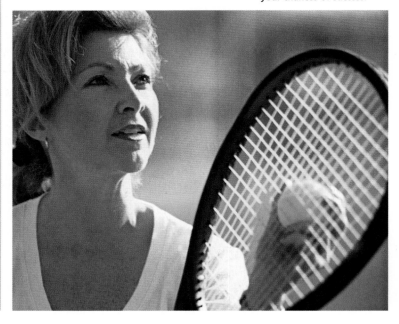

Exercise can offset any weight gain associated with kicking the habit. And studies show it can boost your chances of success.

Twelve reasons to quit

If you are not sure you're ready to throw those cigarettes away, you need to persuade yourself that the benefits are worth the effort. The first step is to consider the benefits. With smoking, that shouldn't be difficult. Consider these incentives.

1 You'll live longer. Men who quit before the age of 39 add an average five years to their lives. Women gain an additional three years. Even smokers who wait until their 60s to quit live an extra year longer.

2 You'll have more energy and stamina to do the things you enjoy.

3 You'll look better. Smoking stains the teeth and causes premature wrinkling and drying of the skin.

4 You'll be healthier. Smoking is the leading cause of lung cancer, emphysema and bronchitis.

5 When you light up, you expose the people you love to the hazards of passive smoking. It is thought that at least 3,600 people die annually in the UK from exposure to secondhand smoke at home; another 700 from exposure at work. Passive smoking is believed to cause as many as 16,900 deaths a year in people aged over 65.

6 Smoking reduces the ratio of LDL ('bad' cholesterol) to HDL ('good' cholesterol) in your blood.

7 Smoking generates free radicals, unstable molecules that oxidize deposits of cholesterol on the lining of blood vessel walls, making them more likely to rupture and cause heart attacks.

8 Nicotine raises blood pressure by 15 to 25mm mercury after you inhale a cigarette.

9 Smoking increases the risk of the blood clots that can cause heart attacks.

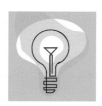

LOOKING AHEAD

Is smoking a cigar safer than smoking cigarettes?

Martin Dunn, counsellor with additional training in smoking cessation, working for Quit, the charity whose aim is to help people to stop smoking.

'Both can kill you. Some cigar smokers think that smoking cigars is safer than cigarettes because most cigar smokers don't inhale. But surveys show that 10 per cent of cigar puffers do inhale. Even those who don't inhale, breathe in plenty of secondhand smoke. Plus they swallow toxic substances from cigar smoke, which include more nicotine, benzine, lead-nitrogen oxides and other harmful chemicals than cigarette smoke contains.

'People who smoke cigars don't tend to light up as often as cigarette smokers. But they face the same risks as cigarette smokers of heart disease, chronic pulmonary disease and cancers of the mouth, oesophagus and lungs.'

One UK study found that compared to non-smokers, cigar smokers have a significantly higher risk of stroke, major coronary heart disease (CHD) and premature death from cardiovascular and other causes. The study also found a sigificantly higher incidence of smoking-related cancers.

10 In men, smoking can lead to impotence.

11 Smoking narrows the blood vessels, increasing the likelihood that coronary arteries already constricted by atherosclerosis will become so obstructed that angina or a heart attack results.

12 If you smoke, your children are more likely to do so, too.

Plan how you are going to quit

When you decide you're ready to stop, make an appointment with your doctor to discuss your decision. This is because studies have shown that person-to-person tobacco dependence counselling, either one-to-one or through a group, boosts your chances of success. Your doctor can should be able to refer you to one of the NHS smoking cessation clinics. If that's not possible, then he or she will recommend one of the nicotine replacement therapies.

At the moment there are at least six forms of nicotine replacement. They include patches, nasal sprays, inhalers, gum, lozenges and microtabs (small tablets that you place under your tongue). The nicotine gum, lozenges, microtabs, nasal spray and inhalator deliver a high dose quickly, so that you can respond to a craving with a 'quick fix'. If you used to smoke steadily through the day, a patch may suit you better. The inhalator may be helpful if you miss the 'hand to mouth' action of smoking. Analysis conducted in 2000 found that people on nicotine-replacement therapy increased their odds of quitting by 70 per cent.

SMOKING-CESSATION AIDS

These aids can significantly boost your chances of quitting. All of them have potential (usually mild) side effects. You must have stopped smoking completely before starting medication.

MEDICATION	POSSIBLE SIDE EFFECTS	DURATION	AVAILABILITY
Sustained-release bupropion (Zyban)	Insomnia,dry mouth maintenance,up to 6 months	7 to 12 weeks;	Prescription only
Nicotine gum	Mouth soreness, indigestion	At least 3 months	Over-the-counter
Nicotine inhalator	Mouth and throat irritation	Up to 3 months	Prescription only
Nicotine lozenge	Sore throat, dizziness, indigestion	12 weeks to 6months	Over-the-counter
Nicotine nasal spray	Nasal irritation	Up to 8 weeks	Prescription only
Microtabs	Dizziness, headache, nausea	Up to 12 weeks	Prescription only
Nicotine patch	Local skin reaction	Up to 12 weeks	Prescription only

Can hypnosis or acupuncture help?

Hypnotic suggestion has been used for decades to help smokers to give up cigarettes. But even the experts can't agree on whether it works.

On the positive side, researchers at Ohio State University interviewed 452 people who had participated in a group-hypnotherapy smoking-cessation programme. Five to 15 months after attending the single-day programme, 22 per cent of the participants said they had not smoked in the preceding month. Hypnosis, the researchers concluded, offers a reasonable alternative to other smoking-cessation methods.

But not everyone is convinced. When researchers from the University of Leicester analysed nine studies that used hypnosis to enable smokers to stop smoking, they found no evidence that this method helped.

The verdict on acupuncture is just as mixed. The ancient healing practice involves the insertion of small needles just below the surface of the skin at specific sites on the body, such as the ear lobes, chest or arms.

Some studies have shown real benefit. At the University of Oslo, in Norway, researchers randomly divided 46 men and 39 women into two groups. One group received acupuncture at locations on their bodies traditionally identified as antismoking points. The other received a placebo treatment: needles inserted at random locations not associated with addiction. Volunteers in both groups reduced the number of cigarettes smoked each day. But 31 per cent of the smokers receiving genuine acupuncture managed to quit successfully during the course of the study. Not a single one of the smokers who received fake acupuncture was able to give up cigarettes for good.

In the UK, a 1998 study showed similar positive results. In a group of 78 smokers, 12.5 per cent of those in the acupuncture group had successfully quit after six months compared with none in the control group.

But not all the reports are encouraging. In 2001, researchers in Germany reviewed 39 studies of the benefits of acupuncture. They found no convincing evidence that genuine acupuncture was any better than sham acupuncture in smoking cessation.

What's the verdict? If you're determined to give acupuncture or hypnosis a try, look for a practitioner associated with a local hospital or clinic. That way you're more likely to find someone with bona fide credentials. If you haven't stopped smoking within a month, it's time to choose another approach.

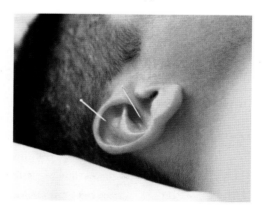

Some people swear by these approaches, claiming they've helped them to stop smoking, even after just one session. Others say they're bogus. What's the real truth?

Changing smoking's image

In May 2004, the British Heart Foundation reported that its potent image of the fatty cigarette dripping artery-clogging goo was proving remarkably effective. In one survey 83 per cent of smokers said that the ad had made them rethink their habit.

Stuart Austin, 38, from Richmond, who gave up after seeing it, said, 'I found the advert so disgusting that it was no real effort to give up. I found that I physically couldn't touch another cigarette. Just thinking of all that fat inside my arteries made me feel sick.'

Back in 1989, the state of California's Tobacco Control Program countered advertising images of smoking as glamorous and sexy with images of the real costs of smoking. In one famous ad the Marlboro man is seen puffing on a drooping cigarette – referring to the fact that smoking can cause impotence in men. In another, tobacco-company executives meet in a smoke-filled room, plotting ways to find new customers to replace those who died from smoking. According to a 2001 survey, a million fewer Californians smoke as a result of the Program's efforts.

These approaches can work for you. Create a mental image of smoking as dirty and unhealthy for you and the people around you. Associate cigarettes with those executives in that smoke-filled room who have used every trick in the book to hook you onto this addictive and potentially lethal product. Don't let them keep you enslaved to nicotine.

View smoking as a dirty, dangerous habit, and you'll be less tempted to light up.

The sixth smoking-cessation aid is a prescription medication called Zyban (bupropion). It was first used to treat depression. Clinical trials in the USA found it helped smokers to quit. It appears to work by acting on the pathways in the brain that are responsible for nicotine addiction. It should reduce the desire to smoke and help to relieve the unpleasant symptoms associated with stopping. When starting bupropion, most people take one tablet a day for the first six days, then two tablets a day for the rest of the course, which usually lasts eight weeks. It will be prescribed by your doctor.

It should not be used by pregnant women, people who suffer from fits, anorexia nervosa, bulimia, kidney or liver problems. It is best not to use bupropion at the same time as other nicotine replacement products, either.

Countdown to quitting

Once you've talked to your doctor, it's time to prepare for the big day when you'll give up tobacco. Most experts recommend spending a week or so getting ready. (If you're a very heavy smoker, however, you may want to wean yourself down to a packet a day before you try to quit. One way to do this is by smoking one less cigarette each day.) During this preparation period, you stiffen your resolve and gain skills that will help you to stop for good.

Five days before quitting

● Fill out the Commit to quit form on page 66. Stick it on your refrigerator or in your office, or both.

● Tell friends and family that you've decided to quit.

● To celebrate your decision, smoke one less cigarette today than you did yesterday.

● If you've decided to use Zyban, begin taking the medication as directed by your doctor.

● Make an appointment with your dental hygienist to have your teeth cleaned on quit day minus one.

Four days before quitting

● Start keeping a daily record of when and why you smoke. To help yourself to remember, fold the sheet of paper that you use for the log around your packet of cigarettes and secure it with a rubber band so that you have to unfold the paper to get a cigarette. Be sure to record things that trigger smoking, such as meals, certain surroundings or stressful situations.

● Make a list of habits or routines you may need to change to make quitting easier. For example, if you usually sit down to have a cigarette with your morning coffee, consider drinking your coffee on the go instead or even switching to tea, instead. Breaking the routine helps.

TROUBLESHOOTING TIP

To boost your chances of success, pick a good time to quit. Holidays, difficult periods at work and other stressful circumstances can weaken your resolve. Choose a time when you feel you can really focus on your goal.

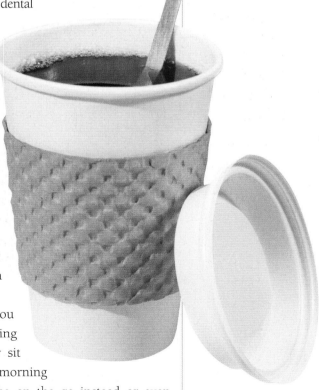

Commit to quit

Use this form to put your commitment to quitting – and your strategies to make it happen – in writing. Stick it up where you'll see it often.

I commit to quit on _____ (date).

My top five strategies for quitting [including any medications you intend to use to help you quit] are:

- _____
- _____
- _____
- _____
- _____

I anticipate the most difficult times will be:

- _____
- _____
- _____
- _____
- _____

Three people I can turn to for support are:

- _____
- _____
- _____

My three most important reasons for quitting are:

- _____
- _____
- _____

Signed:

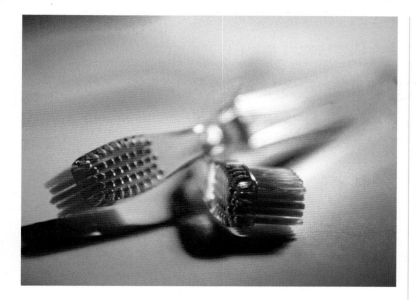

- Plan alternative ways to relax, including simple deep-breathing exercises or even a humorous website you can log onto at any time.
- Think of items you can hold in your hand instead of a cigarette, like a pencil, a chopstick or a squeezable stress-relief ball.
- Smoke one less cigarette than you did yesterday.
- Brush your teeth four times today and appreciate how clean and fresh your mouth tastes afterwards.

Three days before quitting

- Write down the names of two or three people you can call on when you need some moral support – and let them know they're on your list.
- Think of something you can buy yourself as a reward with the money you save on cigarettes over the next two weeks.
- Continue brushing your teeth four times a day.
- Smoke one less cigarette today than you did yesterday.

Two days before quitting

- Buy nicotine gum or whichever smoking-cessation aid you've decided to use, if you've decided to use one.
- Wash your clothes or get them dry-cleaned to get rid of that nasty cigarette smell.
- Brush your teeth four times a day.
- Smoke one less cigarette today than you did yesterday.

TROUBLESHOOTING TIP

The immediate need for a cigarette can seem overpowering, but cravings typically persist only for about 5 minutes. The trick is to outlast them. When a craving hits, make a phone call – even if it's just to make an appointment or check your bank balance. Chances are the urge will subside by the time you hang up.

One day before quitting

● At the end of the day, throw away all cigarettes and matches and put everything that reminds you of smoking – ashtrays and lighters – out of sight. Remove the lighter from your car.

● Remind friends, family and co-workers that tomorrow is the day you plan to quit.

● Stock up on peppermints, gum, pumpkin seeds, carrot sticks or whatever else might distract you from smoking.

● Go to your dental hygienist and have your teeth cleaned. Keep them clean by brushing them several times during the day.

● Smoke one less cigarette today than you did yesterday.

The day you will quit

● Stay busy. Be sure to plan enough activities today to keep yourself well and truly distracted.

● Alter your routine to avoid situations in which you would normally smoke. If you usually smoked during your lunch hour, take a brisk walk instead. If possible, avoid the person with whom you used to share your cigarette break.

● Remind yourself of your list of things to do when the craving strikes and be prepared to do them.

● Avoid alcohol if it makes you want to smoke.

● Celebrate your first smoke-free day by treating yourself to something you really want.

● If you don't manage to get through the whole day without a cigarette, don't despair. Quitting is an on-going project, not a one-time event.

▼ Key finding

A programme of vigorous exercise can help women to both quit smoking and keep weight off, a 1999 study found. Researchers divided 281 sedentary smokers into two groups. One group enrolled in a smoking-cessation programme. The other combined the same programme with three supervised exercise sessions a week. Those in the exercise group were more than twice as likely to be smoke-free at the end of 12 months. They had also gained less weight than the non-exercisers.

Taming temptation

You'll need plenty of willpower – and a little ingenuity – to resist the desire to light up. Think of it as a creative challenge. To get you started, here are 11 tried-and-trusted temptation fighters.

▎**Go somewhere else** Avoid places that serve as triggers for smoking. When the urge to smoke strikes, escape to a smoke-free environment like a library, church, museum or shop. Head to the

REAL PEOPLE, REAL WISDOM

The power of persistence

'It's been a rocky road', says Geoffrey van den Heedon, 61, an Elvis impersonator from Newport who used to smoke 80 cigarettes a day even while performing to crowds at packed-out gigs.

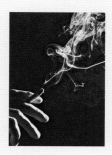

Geoffrey started smoking at the age of 12 and was addicted by the time he was 14. 'It was the thing to do,' he said. 'All the family smoked'.

Although he loved playing the guitar, he needed to earn a living and so became a butcher. All of a sudden he had some money, and after starting on 10 cigarettes a day, it soon got to 15 and then 20.

'When I was in my thirties, I was a landlord in Bristol. Life was fine – it was going on for ever.' Then his mum, dad and brother died within 12 months, all of smoking-related diseases. 'It was too much to cope with. I spiralled down and hit rock-bottom. My voice was suffering; I had chest pains and I was coughing up blood.' My doctor warned me that, with my family history, smoking could kill me.

One Sunday morning after his Elvis Tribute act, he realised he'd smoked 80 cigarettes the day before. Enough was enough. He went to his doctor who prescribed nicotine patches.

He started a diary in which his day-by-day progress was recorded meticulously. Every time he was tempted, he looked in his diary and thought about the money he'd saved. 'Quitting has made the biggest difference in my life – the way I feel when I sing and the energy I have. Before I couldn't walk 100 yards; now I walk half a mile to the pool, swim 30 lengths and walk home. What an achievement that is for me!'

With the money he saved, Geoffrey fulfilled his dream when he went to visit Elvis's Graceland, in Memphis, Tennessee, last year. 'I'm a free spirit, now!' he laughs. 'Life has never been better. Smoking is the devil in disguise.'

cinema for the ultimate distraction, and you'll be sure of about two hours without a cigarette.

2 Nibble carrots or celery sticks Crunching on either not only helps satisfy the oral craving but also gives you something to do with your hands.

3 Chew gum Many smokers find chewing gum satisfies the urge to put a cigarette between their lips. If you're worried about weight gain, choose a sugar-free gum or peppermints.

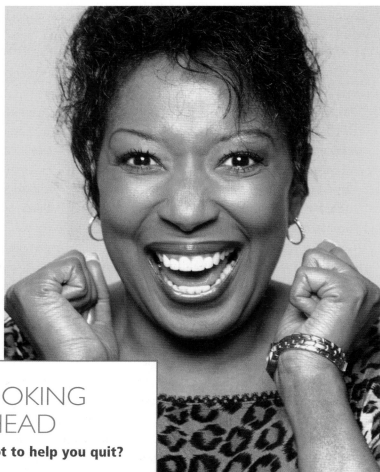

LOOKING AHEAD

A shot to help you quit?

Cambridge-based British pharmaceutical company Xenova is exploring the possibility of a vaccine to free smokers from nicotine addiction. Researchers say that the first phase of the clinical trials showed good results and that the immunizations could be used to block or reduce the intake of nicotine into the brain, thus reducing its addictive power. An anti-smoking vaccine could help to prevent adolescent puffers from becoming confirmed smokers. It could also help to keep former smokers from relapsing.

4 Get up and get moving Take a walk around the block, hop on your bike or exercise cycle and work up a sweat. Exercise can take the edge off nicotine cravings and also help to keep off unwanted pounds. Joining a gym will give you a non-smoking place to go and something new to focus on.

5 Eat several small meals instead of one big one Eating mutes the oral craving for cigarettes. If you're eating or drinking, you have less of an urge to smoke. Also, having smaller meals and eating more frequently keeps your blood sugar levels steady so that you don't overeat, which can help you to avoid gaining weight.

6 Call a friend Don't be ashamed to say, 'Help! I'm weakening'. Good friends or loving relatives will do all they can to encourage or distract you.

7 Practise breathing exercises Find a quiet spot to sit, close your eyes and relax by inhaling and exhaling slowly a dozen times. Breathe from your abdomen, not your chest. Doing this can help to short-circuit the urge to light up.

8 Take a warm shower or bath This is an excellent way to release tension and overcome the craving for cigarettes. Smoking and water don't mix.

9 Wash the dishes Instead of loading the dishwasher and then lighting up after a meal, wash the dishes by hand, to keep your hands busy and your cravings under control.

10 Take up a hobby or develop a new craft Keeping your hands busy will make you less likely to reach for a cigarette.

11 Brush your teeth The fresh clean taste in your mouth may discourage you from polluting it with cigarette smoke.

If at first you don't succeed...

You're not alone. Most long-term smokers try to quit several times before they succeed. Remember that every attempt you make brings you one step closer to your goal. If you do have a lapse, remind yourself that giving in to the urge to smoke a cigarette once or even twice doesn't mean you've failed completely. Too often, people who are trying to make any kind of lasting change in their lives have an all-or-nothing attitude. If they can't kick the habit once and for all, they consider themselves defeated. That kind of thinking turns a momentary slip into a full-scale collapse.

If you falter along the way, don't panic. Instead:

- Remember your three top reasons for wanting to quit.
- Think about what made you smoke that cigarette.
- Write down at least two strategies that will help you to overcome this obstacle next time you encounter it (look back at your Commit to quit form for ideas).
- Set a new quitting date within the coming week.
- Tell at least two friends or family members about your resolution to try again.

The quicker you get back in the game, the better your chances of quitting for good – and the sooner you'll begin to enjoy the benefits of a smoke-free life.

You don't have to go it alone

All kinds of resources out there are devoted to helping you to quit smoking. For more information, check out:

✔ Quit Smoking Helpline
0800 002200
www.quit.org.uk

✔ NHS Smoking Helpline
0800 169 0 169
www.giveupsmoking.co.uk

✔ ASH (Action on Smoking and Health)
www.ash.org.uk

✔ British Heart Foundation Smoking Helpline
0800 169 1 900
www.bhf.org.uk/smoking

5

Heart-healthy eating

The old advice for eating sensibly for your heart has been replaced by a new message: not all fat is bad for your heart. Some of it, such as that found in olive or rapeseed oil and oil-rich fish, is actually good for you. Many foods once banished from a healthy diet, such as nuts and avocados, are now back on the menu. The emphasis has shifted from what you shouldn't eat to what you can and should enjoy – delicious foods that help to protect your heart.

Wholegrain cereals, ripe berries, rich dark breads, salmon, tuna, lean meats, luscious tomatoes, savoury onions, bright orange carrots, fresh leafy greens, even a glass of your favourite wine – they're all part of a diet that's as great tasting as it is good for your heart. So enjoy your food because a healthy diet for your heart is not about deprivation – it's about eating well.

The secrets of a healthy diet

If, like many people in the UK, you greet the latest dietary advice with a pinch of salt, it's no wonder. Nutrition recommendations have made some confusing U-turns in recent years. One day the experts tell us to eat a low-fat, high-carbohydrate diet; the next, it seems, they warn that too many carbohydrates may be dangerous. For years we were told that margarine is a better choice than butter. Then came the news that some types of margarine contain artery-clogging fats. Meanwhile, dozens of new titles crowd bookshop shelves every year, each one claiming to reveal, at long last, the secret of a healthy diet.

The real secret is this: the basics of a heart-healthy diet aren't complicated. And despite the highly publicized reversals, they are rock solid and backed by leading heart and nutrition experts in the UK and abroad. They boil down to just five pieces of advice:

1. Replace saturated fat with unsaturated fat whenever you can.
2. Go easy on foods high in cholesterol.
3. Eat at least five servings of fruit and vegetables a day.
4. Eat plenty of foods made with whole grains.
5. Keep your calorie intake under control.

> *... a healthy diet for your heart is not about deprivation – it's about eating well.*

Ways to cut back on saturated fat

✔ Choose leaner cuts of meat

✔ Remove fat from raw meat whenever possible

✔ Aim to eat smaller meat portions

✔ Add beans in place of some of the meat ino favourite dishes such as shepherd's pie or stews

✔ Substitute low-fat yoghurt for cream

✔ Change your milk to semi-skimmed or skimmed

✔ Enjoy sorbet or low-fat frozen yoghurt instead of ice cream

In this chapter, you will find out how to turn that advice into a satisfying way of eating that won't leave you hungry or longing for something forbidden. It isn't difficult. In fact, many of the world's most cherished traditional cuisines, from Italian pastas and Moroccan couscous to Chinese stir-fries and Mexican rice dishes, follow these simple concepts. Find out how delicious they can be.

Good fat, bad fat

Fat has a bad name. It's very high in calories. Gram for gram, it has more than twice the calories of carbohydrates and has become synonymous with clogged arteries. For years, slashing fat has been considered a priority when it comes to improving your diet.

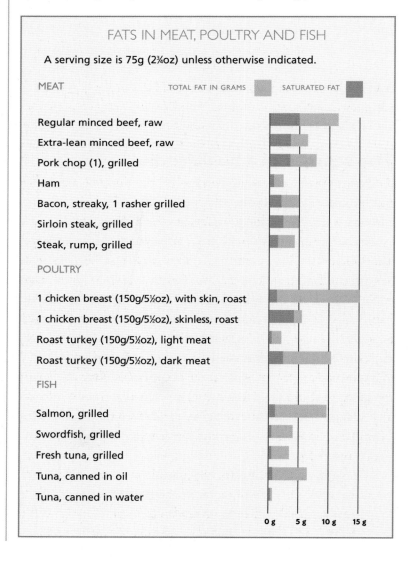

FATS IN MEAT, POULTRY AND FISH

A serving size is 75g (2¾oz) unless otherwise indicated.

MEAT   TOTAL FAT IN GRAMS ◼   SATURATED FAT ◼

Regular minced beef, raw
Extra-lean minced beef, raw
Pork chop (1), grilled
Ham
Bacon, streaky, 1 rasher grilled
Sirloin steak, grilled
Steak, rump, grilled

POULTRY

1 chicken breast (150g/5½oz), with skin, roast
1 chicken breast (150g/5½oz), skinless, roast
Roast turkey (150g/5½oz), light meat
Roast turkey (150g/5½oz), dark meat

FISH

Salmon, grilled
Swordfish, grilled
Fresh tuna, grilled
Tuna, canned in oil
Tuna, canned in water

0 g   5 g   10 g   15 g

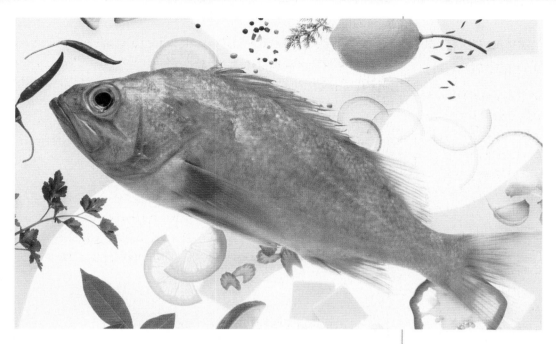

But now we know that not all fat is created equal. Study after study has shown that one kind of fat is particularly dangerous to your arteries, and that's saturated fat, the kind found in fatty cuts of meat, cheese, butter and other high-fat dairy products. When researchers look at different diets around the world, they find that the higher the amount of saturated fat people consume, the higher the rate of heart disease.

Another kind of fat, the unsaturated variety, actually turns out to be beneficial to your heart. Unsaturated fat is found in vegetable oils, oil-rich fish, nuts, seeds, avocados and olive oil. The more unsaturated fat the diet contains, the lower the risk of heart disease.

How can one fat be bad for you and another good? The answer has to do with what happens in your body after you consume them. Saturated fat triggers the production of artery-clogging LDL cholesterol. The more saturated fat you eat, the higher your LDL and total cholesterol numbers are likely to be. Unsaturated fat, on the other hand, keeps LDL levels down and boosts artery-friendly HDL cholesterol. Unsaturated fat has been shown to reduce the risk of erratic heartbeats, and it helps to prevent blood clots, which can trigger heart attacks.

One way to distinguish saturated from unsaturated fat is to think about the source of each of them. Saturated fat is found mostly in animal foods: meat and high-fat dairy products. Unsaturated fat comes mainly from plant foods. the only exceptions are palm oil and coconut oil, which are saturated. Saturated fat is usually solid at room temperature (think of bacon grease or butter). Unsaturated fat is typically liquid (think of vegetable oil).

When low-fat diets were first applauded, many nutritionists recommended replacing fats with carbohydrates. Manufacturers responded with new products. Suddenly all kinds of low-fat biscuits and cakes crowded supermarket shelves and the public – believing the nutritionists – bought them. That wasn't such a good

Rate your diet

How healthy is your diet? Answer these 12 questions and circle the number to the right of your answer. When you have finished, add up your score.

How many servings of fruit do you eat on a typical day?
(A serving is 1 apple, banana, orange, or other fruit, or 150ml/5fl oz cup of juice)
- 3 or more. 2
- 1–2 1
- 0 0

How many servings of vegetables?
(A serving is 3 heaped tbsp of raw, cooked, frozen or canned vegetables, or 1 dessert bowl of salad)
- 3 or more. 2
- 1–2 1
- 0 0

What kind of milk do you drink?
- Skimmed 3
- Soya. 3
- Don't drink milk 0
- Semi-skimmed 2
- Whole 0

Which of the following do you use most often when cooking?
- Olive oil or rape seed oil 3
- Cholesterol-lowering margarine 3
- Other vegetable oils 2
- Soft margarine 1
- Hard margarine. 0

- Butter. 0
- Vegetable shortening 0

How often do you eat salmon or other fish during a typical week?
- 4 or more times 3
- 2–3 times. 2
- Once 1
- Rarely or never eat fish 0

How often do you eat red meat during a typical week, including hamburgers?
- Rarely or never 3
- 1–2 times. 2
- 3–4 times. 1
- 5 or more times 0

What kind of bread do you prefer?
- Whole grain (wholemeal or granary) . 3
- Don't eat bread 1
- White bread 0

How often do you eat takeaways or ready meals
- Rarely or never 3
- 1–2 a month 2
- 1–2 a week 1
- more than 2 a week 0

idea. Very low-fat, high-carbohydrate diets, scientists have realized, have an undesirable effect on cholesterol. It's true, they may lower total cholesterol levels, but they also lower HDL cholesterol, the good kind. In addition, they raise triglycerides, which have been shown to be a risk factor for heart disease.

Dutch scientists demonstrated the dangers of slashing fat and boosting carbohydrates very clearly when they tested two different eating plans on 48 volunteers. Half the subjects consumed

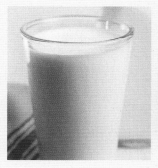 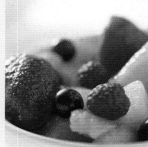 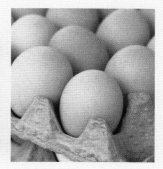

Which of the following foods do you eat frequently (at least twice a week)?
- Brown rice/wholemeal bread 3
- Wholegrain breakfast cereals 3
- Wholegrain pasta 2
- Sugar-coated breakfast cereals 0
- Fried potatoes 0

What do you typically have for dessert?
- Fruit, fresh or canned in
  natural juice 3
- Yoghurt or low-fat fromage frais 2
- Don't eat dessert 2
- Sorbet or fruit canned in syrup 1
- Cake, pie or pastries 0

What is your body mass index, or BMI (see chart on page 131)?
- 18.5–24.9 3
- 25–29.9 1
- 30 or higher 0

Which of the following are you most likely to choose for a snack?
- Fruit 3
- Unsalted nuts 3
- Seeds 3
- Granola bar 2
- Chocolate bar 0
- Crisps 0
- Cookies 0

A score of 34 or more means you're already eating a heart-healthy diet. Keep up the good work, and you'll keep on reaping the benefits.

A score of 25 to 34 means you've made some healthy choices. A few changes can help you to lower your risk of heart disease even further.

A score of 0 to 25 means there is lots of room to improve on your diet. This chapter will show you how.

Ways to replace saturated fat with unsaturated fat

✔ Dip your bread in olive oil instead of using butter

✔ Cook with vegetable oil instead of butter or lard

✔ Use nuts or seeds in stir-fries instead of meat

✔ Add an avocado slice to your sandwich instead of cheese

✔ Try mayonnaise made with rapeseed oil

✔ Avoid shop-bought cakes and biscuits and make your own using vegetable oil instead of butter.

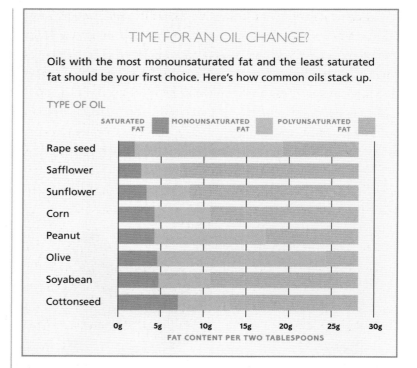

TIME FOR AN OIL CHANGE?

Oils with the most monounsaturated fat and the least saturated fat should be your first choice. Here's how common oils stack up.

TYPE OF OIL

	SATURATED FAT	MONOUNSATURATED FAT	POLYUNSATURATED FAT
Rape seed			
Safflower			
Sunflower			
Corn			
Peanut			
Olive			
Soyabean			
Cottonseed			

0g   5g   10g   15g   20g   25g   30g

FAT CONTENT PER TWO TABLESPOONS

a low-fat, high-carbohydrate diet. The others ate foods low in saturated fat but rich in olive oil, an unsaturated fat. Total cholesterol levels fell in both groups. But among the volunteers on the low-fat, high-carbohydrate diet, HDL levels plummeted, and triglycerides soared.

Such results have convinced many heart experts that the best advice is not to cut total fat but rather to replace saturated fat with unsaturated fat. That's great news if you love good food. Instead of butter, you can use olive and rapeseed oils as both are high in unsaturated fat. Or you can choose a spread made from unsaturated fats. You can also serve plenty of oily fish. Fish oil, in fact, appears to be one of the heart healthiest oils around, being rich in omega-3 fatty acids, which are believed to protect against heart disease.

Long-standing public health advice is that people should eat at least two portions of fish a week, and one of them should be oily fish. The Scientific Advisory Committee on Nutrition recently reported that, on average, people in the UK eat a third of a portion of oily fish a week. Seven out of ten eat none.

Studies have shown that omega-3s lower triglyceride levels. They may also reduce the risk of small blood clots that can lead to heart attacks. Further, fish oil seems to stabilize the heartbeat, lowering the risk of irregular heart rhythms associated with sudden cardiac failure. In the Seven Countries study, which looked at heart disease risk in different populations around the world, researchers found that men who ate no fish had the highest rate of death from coronary artery disease. Those who ate the most fish had the lowest rate.

In recent years new spreads, such as Benecol and Flora Proactiv, have appeared and claim to contain compounds that can reduce cholesterol levels by 10 to 15 per cent by reducing the absorption of cholesterol by the intestine, compelling the liver to remove more harmful LDL cholesterol, thereby reducing LDL levels in the blood.

How low should you go?

Experts agree that it's important to eat less saturated fat. And in the UK they are quite clear on the limits. The British Heart Foundation and the government's advisory committee, the Committee on Medical Aspects of Food and Nutrition Policy (COMA) both agree

Hot topic: Battle of the omegas

There are two forms of unsaturated fat available to us: monounsaturated and polyunsaturated. Olive oil is especially rich in the former. Corn oil and soya bean oil are loaded with the latter. Which is the healthier choice? Both are good for your heart. Some experts suspect there may be an optimum balance between the two, but so far no one agrees on what that may be.

Some researchers think that the balance between two types of polyunsaturated fat matters more. The first, found in sunflower and other oils, is rich in omega-6 fatty acids. The second, found in oily fish, and also flaxseed, walnuts and rapeseed oil are omega-3 fatty acids. The Scientific Advisory Committee on Nutrition recommends that people eat at least two portions of oily fish a week, one of which

should be oily, which would increase their intake of omega-3s from about 0.1g a day to 0.2g a day. This is because, as well as helping to protect the heart, omega-3 fats have anti-inflammatory properties that help to protect against conditions such as rheumatoid arthritis and inflammatory bowel disease. They are also believed to reduce the risk of certain types of cancer. A simple way to add omega-3s is to eat more fish and cook with rapeseed oil.

But some researchers aren't convinced that it's worth worrying about balancing omega-3s and omega-6s. Nor do they think you need to bother about monounsaturated fat vs polyunsaturated fat. The real key is eating less saturated fat, by consuming fewer foods loaded with saturated fat and by replacing saturated with unsaturated fat.

Meals for all seasons

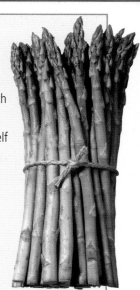

One of the joys of locally grown fruits and vegetables is their seasonality. Ripe pears come around only once a year. Tender asparagus arrives in spring. Late summer brings luscious tomatoes. By November the markets are full of pumpkins and apples. Let the season's produce inspire your meals. When the first local tomatoes appear at farmer's markets, serve them sliced with olive oil and vinegar or roughly chopped in your favourite pasta. If you like spicy greens, make a salad with watercress or rocket. On a sultry summer day, cool yourself down with chilled gazpacho, a cold soup made with finely diced tomatoes, onions, green peppers and parsley. Enjoy pumpkin soup and baked apples on a winter's night.

> **Replacing just 5 per cent of saturated fat with unsaturated ... can reduce your risk of heart attack by about 40 per cent.**

that about 35 per cent of calories in our daily diet should come from fat and 10 per cent or less should come from saturated fat. Interestingly, some US researchers think that's far too much total fat. University of California's Dr Dean Ornish, for instance, is convinced that the best way to prevent heart attacks is to slash total fat to less than 10 per cent of calories and virtually eliminate saturated fat. In his landmark Lifestyle Heart Trial, Dr Ornish tested such an ultra-low-fat diet – one that all but banished oil, meat and dairy products – in heart attack survivors. The findings suggested that a very low-fat diet, combined with exercise and stress reduction, might even clear out arteries clogged with plaque, reversing heart disease.

Other researchers maintain that the healthiest diet is one with as much as 40 per cent of daily calories from fat – as long as it's unsaturated. The model is the Mediterranean diet. It's not low in total fat but most of the fat comes from olive oil, seafood and nuts. That, some scientists now think, makes all the difference.

In fact, when researchers looked at data from the Nurses' Health Study, they found no link at all between total fat consumption and risk of heart disease or heart attack. What did matter was the kind of fat. Women who consumed more unsaturated fat were less likely to develop heart disease than women who consumed more saturated fat. Replacing just 5 per cent of saturated fat with unsaturated, the researchers calculated – switching from butter to olive oil, for instance, and favouring fish over beef – can reduce your risk of heart attack by about 40 per cent.

The Mediterranean model

Another study provided further evidence in favour of fats. The Lyon Diet Heart Study, conducted in France, looked at 605 men and women who had survived a first heart attack. Some were asked to follow a diet with about 30 per cent of calories from fat. The others were put on a higher-fat Mediterranean diet rich in unsaturated fats. It included more bread, vegetables, fish, poultry and fruit, less red meat, no cream and a special margarine made with unsaturated oil containing omega-3 fatty acids (also found in fish). After two and a half years, the investigators were ordered to stop the trial because the risk of death among people on the Mediterranean diet was so much lower than the risk for people in the first group – about 70 per cent less – that the ethics and safety committee wanted everyone to be offered the Mediterranean diet.

How much total fat should your diet include? If you've already been diagnosed with atherosclerosis or coronary artery disease, talk this question over with your doctor. If your HDL levels are lower than ideal, a diet higher in unsaturated fat may make sense. If you're trying to lose weight, you may do better on a lower-fat diet. The essential thing is to find ways to reduce saturated fat. As mentioned earlier, the British Heart Foundation and the Scientific Advisory Committee on Nutrition recommend no more than 10 per cent of calories from saturated fat; if you've been diagnosed with heart disease, you may want to cut it back further to 7 per cent.

A hidden danger: trans fat

Not long ago, researchers discovered another kind of fat that poses a serious heart danger: hydrogenated fat, also called trans fat. Trans fat is a man-made concoction, first devised by food chemists more than a century ago. By tinkering with hydrogen molecules, they discovered that they could turn liquid vegetable oil into a solid. The result: a vegetable oil that could be used instead of butter or lard. The first margarine was born. Soon these vegetable fats took their place in almost every cook's cupboard. Hydrogenated fats also showed up in all kinds of snacks and processed foods. Unfortunately, it turns out that these fats are worse for your arteries than saturated fat, because they raise LDL cholesterol (the bad kind) and drag down HDL cholesterol (the good kind).

10 top sources of omega-3s

1 Mackerel (fresh or frozen)
2 Kipper
3 Fresh tuna
4 Trout
5 Salmon
6 Herring (pickled)
7 Pilchard (canned in tomato sauce)
8 Salmon (canned)
9 Sardines (canned)
10 Swordfish

MILK FACTS

Still drinking full-fat milk? Time to lighten up. The easiest approach is to switch to the next lower level of fat – from whole to semi-skimmed, for instance, or from semi-skimmed to skimmed. It won't take long before skimmed milk tastes as good as the one you were drinking before. And by lowering the fat in the milk you drink, you'll also reduce both cholesterol and calories. Figures below are given for 100ml (3½fl oz) of milk.

TYPE OF MILK	TOTAL FAT	SATURATED FAT	CHOLESTEROL	CALORIES
Whole	3.9%	2.5g	14mg	66
Semi-skimmed	1.6%	1.1g	6mg	46
Skimmed	0.1%	0.3g	3mg	33

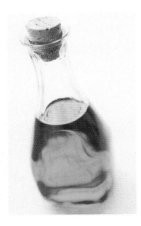

FAST FACT
When you're shopping for olive oil, choose extra virgin. According to Spanish researchers, this form, which is unrefined, is better than others at preventing the oxidation of LDL cholesterol that damages arteries.

Ridding your diet of trans fats isn't easy. They turn up in all kinds of foods, from some types of margarine and vegetable shortenings to processed foods. The fast-food industry uses hydrogenated fats for deep-frying everything from chicken nuggets to French fries. Avoiding all this artery-clogging fat is not easy, especially as trans fats don't have to be included in the nutritional information provided on a food label. If you are eating in a fast-food restaurant, go easy on fried foods. Better still, choose the healthy option that many are offering now. And instead of snacking on potato crisps, have a handful of nuts instead.

Whatever happened to cholesterol?

Remember when dietary cholesterol was public health enemy number one? When it seemed that all we had to do was buy foods marked 'cholesterol free' and we'd never have to worry about heart disease again? Nutritionists say it is still a good idea to limit your intake of dietary cholesterol if you have high blood cholesterol levels. But the obsession with dietary cholesterol has given way to a focus on saturated fat.

This is because the amount of cholesterol that you consume isn't directly linked to cholesterol in your blood. When you eat cholesterol-rich foods, the cholesterol they contain ends up in your liver. There, it slows the liver's production of a protein that helps to remove LDL cholesterol from the blood. So in theory, the more cholesterol you eat, the higher the level of LDL in your blood.

But in reality, the connection is a bit more complicated. The liver itself manufactures cholesterol, which is used to build cell walls, make hormones and fulfil other important functions in the body. About 20 per cent of cholesterol comes directly from the diet and the liver produces the other 80 per cent. To keep blood-cholesterol levels steady, the liver reacts to the cholesterol coming in from food. The more we eat, the less it churns out. That feedback mechanism helps to keep cholesterol levels relatively stable.

Kinks in the process

In some people – possibly as many as one in five, the feedback mechanism doesn't work efficiently and the liver produces too much LDL cholesterol. (A healthy target LDL cholesterol level is under 3mmol/l.) The amount that diet influences cholesterol levels varies considerably and is probably an inherited characteristic. But if your LDL levels are too high, reducing the amount of cholesterol that you consume from food becomes a little more significant. Total blood cholesterol readings above 6mmol/l are considered high. The amount of cholesterol present in the blood is generally between 3.6mmol/l and 7.8mmol/l. On average, men in this country have a level of 5.5mmol/l and women a level of 5.6mmol/l. Government health advice suggests a target cholesterol level of under 5mmol/l.

Foods that are high in cholesterol

Cholesterol is not found in large amounts in many foods, except in eggs and in offal such as liver and kidneys. The cholesterol in these foods does not usually make a great contribution to your blood cholesterol level, but it is probably wise to limit eggs to about three a week.

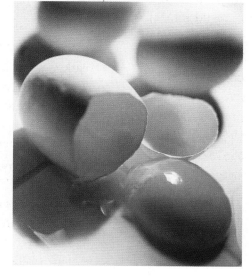

But if you need to reduce your cholesterol level and get that figure down below 5mmol/l, it is much more important to reduce the total amount of fat you eat and to change the types of fat you eat. The more saturated fat you consume, the greater risk you will have of higher blood cholesterol. Medical experts have even produced a formula for it: each 1 per cent decrease in calories from saturated fats in the diet produces a 0.078mmol/l decrease in blood cholesterol.

10 foods rich in antioxidants

1 Spinach
2 Blueberries
3 Strawberries
4 Kale
5 Broccoli
6 Brussels sprouts
7 Cranberries
8 Prunes
9 Tea
10 Grape juice

The rainbow connection

How colourful is your diet? If it's bright with greens, reds, yellows and oranges, you are probably eating the recommended five or more servings of fruits and vegetables a day. But most of us aren't. And that's bad, because these foods are loaded with antioxidants – potent substances that fight cancer, head off heart disease and may protect against a variety of other chronic illnesses, from diabetes to macular degeneration. They do this by blocking damage caused by unstable oxygen molecules known as free radicals. Such damage speeds up the process that turns artery-clogging cholesterol into potentially deadly plaques on vessel walls. Research suggests that oxidation may also be the culprit in Alzheimer's disease.

The more fruits and vegetables you eat, the more protection you get. In fact, you'll find the richest array of antioxidants – from vitamin A to zeaxanthin – in the fruit and vegetable aisles of your shop. While the official advice is to eat at least 5 servings of fruits and vegetables a day, some research suggests the optimal number of these low-fat, high-fibre foods may be as high as 10.

Leafy green vegetables are also loaded with the B vitamin folate (the word comes from 'foliage'). So are citrus fruits. A growing body of evidence suggests that a diet rich in folate helps to keep homeo-cysteine levels from rising, which may help to reduce the risk of heart disease. A recent study found that plenty of folate in the diet can prevent arteries from reclogging after heart-bypass surgery.

A diet rich in fruits and vegetables can head off strokes as well as heart attacks, according to a 1999 report in the *Journal of the American Medical Association.* Scientists found that people who consumed around six servings of fruits and vegetables a day were 30 per cent less likely to have a stroke during the 14-year investigation than those who rarely ate fruit and vegetables. The best protection appeared to come from leafy green cruciferous vegetables like broccoli and from cauliflower, citrus fruit and fruit juice – all abundant sources of fibre.

Fibre for your heart

Something all vegetables and fruits have in common is that they contain fibre – that part of plant foods that the body can't digest. Fibre comes in two basic types. The insoluble kind passes through the digestive tract unchanged. The soluble kind dissolves to form a gummy substance in the intestines.

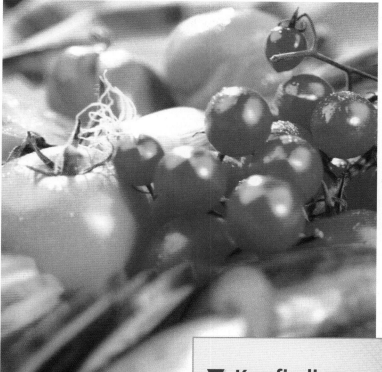

▼ Key finding

Scientists found that volunteers who consumed more than 24g of fibre a day were 50 per cent less likely to develop high blood pressure than those who consumed less than 12g every day.

Both types are important to both heart, and general, health. In the small intestine, soluble fibre slows the absorption of glucose into the bloodstream which helps to keep blood-sugar and insulin levels from rising too fast. That, in turn, can lower your risk of Type 2 diabetes and coronary artery disease. Large amounts of soluble fibre can also trap cholesterol and help to remove it from the body as waste. Insoluble fibre slows down the progress of food through the intestines, helping to prevent constipation.

Although there's no UK legislation governing fibre claims, the Food Standards Agency recommends that anything labelled as a 'source' of fibre should contain 3g of fibre per 100g/ml or 'at least 3g in the reasonable expected daily intake of the food' – that is, the amount that anyone could be expected to eat in a day. If the food is naturally high in fibre, it can be called 'a high-fibre food'. To be able to claim a high-fibre content, the food must contain at least 6g per 100g/ml or at least 6g in a reasonable daily intake.

FAST FACT

In the UK, most people eat far too little fibre – on average, 12g a day or less. Ideally, adults should aim for a daily intake of about 18g, or even a little more.

Foods high in soluble fibre

1 Oats and oat bran
2 Beans and pulses
3 Peas
4 Rice bran
5 Barley
6 Citrus fruits
7 Strawberries

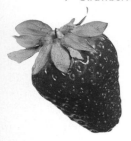

Foods high in insoluble fibre

1   Whole wheat breads
2   Wheat cereals
3   Brown rice
4   Barley & other grains
5   Cabbage
6   Beetroot
7   Carrots
8   Brussels sprouts
9   Turnips
10 Cauliflower

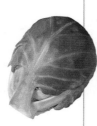

There's plenty of evidence that eating foods rich in fibre offers powerful heart protection. In a 1999 study, researchers found that men and women who consumed the greatest amount of fibre every day had significantly lower blood pressure, triglyceride levels and LDL cholesterol than those who ate the least. They were also less likely to gain weight.

New findings from the Harvard School of Public Health show that every helping of fruit or vegetables you add to your daily menu cuts your heart disease risk by 4 per cent. That may not sound like a lot. But the study, which followed more than 130,000 men and women over a period of 8 to 14 years, found that those who ate the most fruit and vegetables were 20 per cent less likely to get coronary artery disease than those who ate the least.

The UK daily intake of fibre has declined over the past century. One reason is that meat and fatty foods have crowded out fruit, vegetables and whole grain foods from our diets. If you have risk factors for heart disease – a family history of early heart attacks, for instance, or elevated cholesterol – it's important to aim for more than five servings of fruits and vegetables a day – preferably up to ten. It's not too difficult. Here's a suggested day's meal plan.

Breakfast
- 1 glass (150ml/5fl oz) of orange or grapefruit juice
- porridge with raisins and banana slices or berries

Morning snack
- 1 apple or pear

Lunch
- Chicken or turkey sandwich on wholegrain bread with lettuce and tomato
- Reduced-fat coleslaw (3 tablespoons)

Afternoon snack
- Carrot and celery sticks or a glass of tomato juice

Dinner
- Chicken casserole with jacket potato or brown rice
- Side dish of roasted parsnip or carrots
- Leafy green salad

Dessert
- Mixed berries

Total: 4 servings of fruit and 6 servings of vegetables, for a grand total of 10 servings.

Five 'superstar' foods

Almost any food high in fibre, rich in antioxidants or low in saturated fat is good for your heart. But some foods offer special benefits. Here are five that are worth stocking up on.

I Nuts Once banished from the list of healthy foods because of their high fat content, nuts are suddenly back. Studies show that eating more nuts could actually lower your heart disease risk.

Besides being rich in unsaturated fat, nuts also contain arginine, an amino acid that is needed to make nitric oxide. Nitric oxide, in turn, helps to relax constricted blood vessels and increase blood flow. Nuts are also good sources of vitamin E, an antioxidant. Because nuts are high in calories, enjoy them in moderation, especially if you're trying to lose weight. Almonds and walnuts are particularly heart healthy choices because the fat they contain is almost entirely unsaturated.

2 Lentils Four tablespoons of cooked lentils contain almost 6g of fibre – about a third of the amount experts say we should be getting every day. In a study of 11,629 men and women enrolled in the Scottish Heart Health Study, researchers at the University of Reading looked for links between fibre, antioxidants and cardio-vascular disease. In women, fibre was the most outstanding. A high-fibre diet was found to almost halve the risk of heart disease. Lentils are also an abundant source of folate, which may help to protect arteries by keeping blood levels of homocysteine in check.

WHAT'S IN A NUT?

Nuts are loaded with fat and sometimes salt. But they're no longer banned from a heart-healthy menu because the fat they contain is mostly unsaturated – so they're actually good for your heart.

NUT (28g/1oz)	CALORIES	TOTAL FAT	SATURATED FAT
Almonds	171	15g	1g
Cashews	160	13g	3g
Macadamia	209	22g	3g
Peanuts	158	13g	2.5g
Pistachios	160	13g	1.7g
Walnuts	193	19g	1.6g
Mixed nuts (dry roasted)	170	15g	2.5g

Hot topic: Eating out – but eating sensibly

There's hidden fat in many of the dishes you are offered in restaurants and pubs. Knowing what to avoid is important: it means you can eat healthily and well.

In a restaurant Avoid dishes that contain these words: a la crème, alfredo, au gratin, batter-dipped, battered, béarnaise, béchamel, beurre blanc, breaded, buttered, cordon-bleu, creamed, crispy, en croûte, escalloped, flaky, Florentine, fried, hollandaise, meunière, milanese, pan-fried, puffed, rich, sauté, smothered in and tempura – all fatty options.

Instead, choose: baked, broiled, char-grilled, flame-cooked, grilled, in its own juice, with jus, poached, raw or steamed.

In a pub choose
- Onion soup or carrot and coriander soup, instead of cream of stilton or mushroom soup
- A ham, chicken or tuna sandwich with a salad instead of a ploughman's lunch
- Jacket potato with baked beans or vegetable chilli instead of jacket potato with cheese and coleslaw
- Salmon with new potatoes and peas instead of fish or scampi and chips
- Beef casserole, mashed potato and green vegetables, instead of steak and kidney pie, roast potatoes and gravy
- Fresh fruit salad with ice cream instead of sticky toffee pudding with butterscotch sauce.
- Small portion of apple crumble with custard instead of cheese and biscuits.

In an Indian restaurant choose
- A light starter of pappadums with cucumber raita, instead of oily bhaji, samosa or pakhora
- Chapatti or plain naan bread (made without fat) instead of peshwara, paratha and puris

- Drier dishes, such as tandoori, tikka (although not tikka masala), karia and bhuna instead of creamy korma, masala and dhansak
- Plain boiled rice instead of pilau, biryani or fried rice – all three are very high in fat
- Vegetable dishes not cooked in ghee

In a Chinese restaurant choose
- Won ton soup to start, instead of prawn crackers, sesame prawn rolls and dim sum – unless it is steamed
- Stir-fried, rather than deep-fried dishes. Avoid sweet and sour dishes or crispy fried beef or duck. Have satay and chow mein as a rare treat.
- Steamed or stir-fried vegetables instead of deep fried, which are usually in batter
- Plain rice or noodles instead of fried rice.
Remember that Chinese food can be very salty because soy sauce is used freely.

In a Thai restaurant choose
- Stir-fried chicken or vegetables instead of curries that contain coconut cream.
- Steamed fish instead of fried, which may have been cooked in pork fat
- Plain steamed rice or noodles instead of sticky rice which is higher in fat – and avoid coconut rice as it is high in saturated fat
- Salads, as they are usually fresh and tasty

In an Italian restaurant choose
- Plain bread instead of garlic bread
- Pasta dishes with tomato, onion and basil-based toppings instead creamy cheese sauces or pesto. Carbonara is very high in fat
- Thin-based pizzas with vegetable, chicken, ham or tuna toppings instead of high-fat meat like salami or pepperoni, with lots of cheese
- Vegetarian cannelloni instead of traditional cannelloni, which is very high in saturated fat.

Source: British Heart Foundation *Food should be fun...and healthy!*

3 Tea Tea contains a variety of potent antioxidants that help to protect arteries from damage from free radicals – unstable oxygen molecules that make cholesterol more likely to stick to artery walls. A 1999 study found that women who drank a cup or two of black tea a day were 54 per cent less likely to develop severe atherosclerosis than those who rarely drank tea. The more tea the women drank, the more they benefited. Those who drank four cups a day reduced their risk of atherosclerosis by 69 per cent.

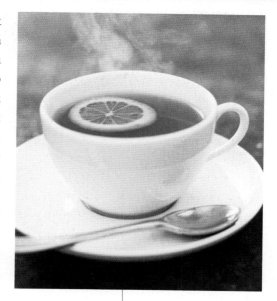

Tea also inhibits blood clotting, which can lead to a heart attack or stroke. Green tea contains more antioxidants than black tea, although both have been shown to lower heart disease risk.

4 Soya Not long ago food manufacturers were given the green light to promote the cholesterol-lowering benefits of soya foods such as tofu and soya milk. A variety of studies have shown that people with elevated cholesterol who add 25g of soya protein to their daily menu can expect to lower total cholesterol by about 9 per cent and LDL cholesterol, the artery-clogging kind, by as much as 15 per cent.

And the benefits may go beyond cholesterol. In Japan and China, where soya is served at almost every meal, rates of breast cancer and prostate cancer are a quarter of what they are in the UK. No one knows for sure that soya is the reason, since Asian diets differ in many ways from ours. But when Japanese researchers compared 1,186 women with breast cancer to 23,163 healthy volunteers, they found that women free of the disease ate tofu much more often than those who developed breast cancer. It may be worth emulating the Japanese and including more tofu in your diet.

5 Avocados Avocados are rich in monounsaturated fat, the same heart-friendly fat found in olive oil and nuts. Gram for gram, they also have more soluble fibre than any other fruit.

In addition, food chemists recently discovered that avocados are bursting with a plant sterol called beta-sitosterol, which helps to prevent cholesterol from being absorbed through the intestines. That means less cholesterol makes its way into your bloodstream. Other fruits and vegetables contain beta-sitosterol, but avocados have more of it than any of them.

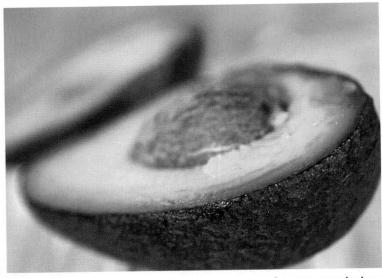

Gram for gram, avocados have more soluble fibre than any other fruit.

When researchers from the Instituto Mexicano del Seguro Social in Mexico asked 45 volunteers to add avocados to their diets for a week, they recorded a significant drop in total cholesterol, artery-choking LDL cholesterol and triglycerides. Those volunteers who had mildly elevated cholesterol saw the biggest benefit: an impressive 17 per cent drop in total cholesterol and a 22 per cent decline in LDL cholesterol. But because they're high in fat, avocados are also high in calories, so don't overdo them.

The whole truth

The more almost any food is processed, the less fibre and fewer nutrients it will contain – and the less protection it will offer your heart. That is especially true of grains. Wheat in its unrefined state has an outer layer rich in fibre, magnesium and vitamins. The germ at its centre is a rich source of additional vitamins, including vitamin E, and unsaturated fats. Refined wheat flour (white flour), on the other hand, has been stripped of most of this goodness. The same is true of white rice (compared with brown rice, which still has its outer bran layer).

▼ Key finding

Research from the University of Cardiff found that people who ate high-fibre breakfast cereals (such as Weetabix or All Bran) every day, reported feeling less tired and stressed than those who ate low-fibre cereals such as cornflakes.

A wild blood-sugar ride

There's another disadvantage to highly processed grains. The carbohydrates in refined flour are much more easily digested and converted into glucose than the more complex carbohydrates in whole-wheat flour. The faster glucose enters the bloodstream, the steeper the rise in blood sugar. You may have heard about the glycaemic index (GI). A food's GI number is determined by how quickly that particular food releases glucose into the system for use by the body. Foods with a high GI number (such as cornflakes and cooked potatoes) are converted into glucose much faster than those with a low GI number (such as porridge oats, basmati rice, beans and pulses).

A diet heavy with foods that rush glucose into the bloodstream can cause a roller-coaster effect because the rise in blood sugar is followed by a parallel rise in insulin, the hormone produced by the pancreas that allows glucose to enter cells, removing it from the bloodstream. If glucose floods into the blood too quickly, the resulting spurt in insulin can drive blood-sugar levels too low. That dip triggers the body's hunger mechanism, which signals us to reach for something to eat. If you choose something rich in simple carbohydrates, you'll find yourself riding a roller coaster of blood-sugar levels throughout the day.

This wild ride, and the sharp hunger pangs that accompany it, can make it tough to maintain your weight. But there are more serious consequences. Spiking blood-sugar and insulin levels add to the risk of Type 2 diabetes, which in turn increases your risk of heart disease – especially if you're overweight. Some researchers believe that the rise in highly processed foods in the UK diet may be one of the chief causes of our epidemic of heart disease.

When researchers analysed the eating habits of 75,000 women over the course of ten years, they found that those who ate the most foods with a high glycaemic index – white bread, white rice, potatoes and

To help to keep your blood sugar steady, enjoy a bowl of muesli or porridge oats instead of cornflakes.

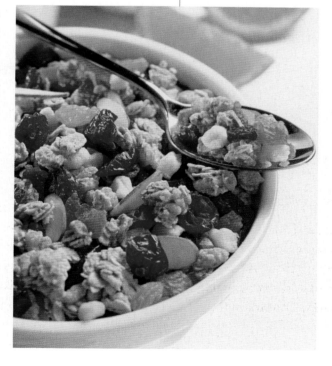

low-fibre cereals – had an 85 per cent greater risk of heart attack than those who ate the least. A surge of sugar into the bloodstream seems to reduce levels of good cholesterol, raise triglycerides and interfere with the body's ability to use insulin.

Getting off the roller coaster

To avoid blood-sugar surges, try to choose foods that are rich in whole grains and complex carbohydrates. In the process, you'll also be taking in more heart-protective fibre and you will get more nutrients and antioxidant vitamins with every mouthful. Here are a few simple tips.

- Start the day with wholegrain cereal. During the winter, sit down to a bowl of old-fashioned porridge (avoid quick and instant varieties, which are highly processed). For cold cereal, try All Bran, Shredded Wheat, muesli and other cereals that list whole wheat as one of the first ingredients.
- Opt for wholemeal breads that include whole wheat, whole oats, whole rye or other whole grain as the main ingredient on the label. Also check the fibre content. Wholemeal foods usually contain plenty of fibre (at least 2 to 3g per serving), unlike highly refined ones.
- Try brown rice instead of white rice. When you cook, look for recipes that use wholemeal flour – or at least allow you to substitute up to half of the white flour with wholemeal.

A toast to good health

The French diet should be a recipe for disaster. Goose and duck-liver patés, creamy sauces and a whole course devoted just to cheese. But the French have some of the lowest rates of heart disease in the world. No one yet knows why, but one reason that they may be able to get away with so many fatty foods is the fact that most of them consume more fruits and vegetables than we do. Another may be their love affair with wine.

The 1994 study on 12,321 British male doctors conducted by Oxford's Radford Infirmary is among many that show moderate consumption of alcohol offers some people real protection against heart disease. Men who drink one or two alcoholic drinks a day have 30 to 40 per cent less risk of heart attack than men who don't drink at all. Women who have an alcoholic drink a day also lower their risk of heart attack by about the same amount.

In 2001, scientists at London's Queen Mary School of Medicine found that polyphenols taken from red wines slowed the test-tube production of endothelin-1, a natural chemical that may help to clog arteries. They found that all types of red wine offered this benefit; Cabernet Sauvignon was most effective. Red grape juice also slowed the production of endothelin-1 but white wine and rosé had no effect at all. Drinking alcohol also raises levels of HDL cholesterol. A study published in the *European Heart Journal* found that wine can open up arteries and increase blood flow.

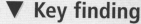

▼ Key finding

The benefits of drinking wine may go beyond heart disease prevention. In a 2004 study, researchers at University College, London, found that moderate wine drinkers have significantly sharper thought-processes than teetotallers. In the latest research, 6,000 civil servants were given tests ranging from verbal and mathematical reasoning problems to test short-term memory. Teetotallers were twice as likely as occasional drinkers to achieve lowest scores. The benefit of alcohol is thought to be linked to its effect on the flow of blood to the brain.

Drinking's downside

Despite all the evidence that moderate consumption of alcohol offers heart protection, many experts are reluctant to recommend that people who don't already drink start imbibing. For one thing, some people are susceptible to

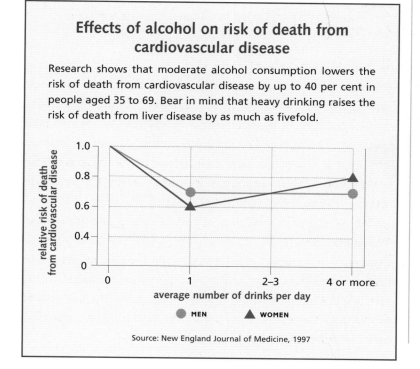

Effects of alcohol on risk of death from cardiovascular disease

Research shows that moderate alcohol consumption lowers the risk of death from cardiovascular disease by up to 40 per cent in people aged 35 to 69. Bear in mind that heavy drinking raises the risk of death from liver disease by as much as fivefold.

relative risk of death from cardiovascular disease

average number of drinks per day

● MEN ▲ WOMEN

Source: New England Journal of Medicine, 1997

alcoholism. And for another, excessive drinking can actually increase the danger of heart disease. It can also cause elevated blood pressure and heart-beat irregularities that can lead to blood clots. Too much alcohol can increase the risk of haemorrhagic stroke (the kind that involves a ruptured blood vessel in the brain). And of course, serious alcoholism can result in liver failure.

Even moderate drinking has raised some other concerns. Several studies have shown that having two alcoholic drinks a day increases a woman's chance of developing breast cancer by 20 to 25 per cent.

Colon cancer rates also appear to be slightly higher in both men and women who drink. New findings suggest that the colon cancer culprit isn't alcohol itself but rather low levels of folic acid in the blood. Alcohol tends to reduce folic-acid levels. As a result, some leading nutritionists recommend that if you drink, you should be sure to take a multivitamin to keep your folic acid levels up.

▼ Key finding

Grape juice may provide some of the same protection you'll get in a glass of wine. Researchers asked 15 patients with clinical signs of cardiovascular disease, including narrowed arteries, to drink a tall glass of grape juice daily.

After 14 days, tests showed a significant reduction in LDL oxidation, a crucial step in the formation of artery-clogging plaque. Ultrasound images showed changes in the artery walls, indicating that blood was flowing more freely.

The heart benefits that alcohol does provide don't apply to everyone. For men over 40, the merits of moderate drinking seem to outweigh any risks. But drinking offers little protection to people in their 20s and 30s, simply because their risk of heart disease is so low to begin with. In the Harvard Nurses' Health Study, the protective effect of alcohol didn't become evident in women until after the age of 50. That makes sense, of course, since it's only after menopause that heart-disease danger climbs steeply in women. In men, the benefits of drinking begin to become evident after the age of 40. Even then, the people who stand to profit most are those with risk factors like elevated cholesterol or a family history of heart problems.

If you already drink, most doctors would simply advise you to make sure that you don't overdo it. If you don't currently drink, don't feel compelled to start. You'll get roughly the same sort of heart benefits from increasing your level of physical activity. And you'll never have to worry if you're fit to drive…

Hot topic: | Cutting back on salt

Should you cut back on salt? For years, experts have disagreed on the answer. Some studies showed that doing so helps to reduce high blood pressure. Others found no benefit.

However, in November 2002, the independent Scientific Advisory Committee on Nutrition, which advises the government, concluded that there is strong evidence of a direct association between salt intake and blood pressure, and that cutting down on salt really could improve this leading risk factor for heart disease. The Food Standards Agency warned that eating too much salt can raise your blood pressure, which triples your risk of developing heart disease, whatever your age.

It recommended that salt consumption should be no more than 6g a day, which is about a teaspoonful. Children should have lower amounts – the younger the child, the less salt should be eaten. Currently, the average British adult consumes about 9.5g of salt a day. In the UK, bread, breakfast cereals, biscuits, cakes and meat products such as bacon, ham and sausages are some of the main sources of salt in the diet.

A significant amount of the salt in our daily diet is hidden in processed foods – up to 75 per cent. In July 2004 the Food Standards Agency carried out a survey that found that many popular food brands contained unhealthy levels of salt. Following a government appeal to major food manufacturers to reduce salt levels, some have since responded by reducing salt content.

Research shows that some people are more salt-sensitive than others, and these people will benefit most by cutting back. But most of us can tame hypertension by cutting down on salt.

Shaking less salt over food is one way, of course. Instead, try using pepper, lemon pepper or other herbs or spices to add flavour, or a product such as LoSalt. Replace salty snacks such as crisps, with unsalted nuts, fruit or carrot sticks.

To bring your salt intake down significantly, however, you'll have to look at the labels of the prepared foods you eat. Many are loaded with salt. Consider this:

- One serving of canned beef ravioli in tomato and meat sauce contains 2.9g salt (1,173mg sodium).
- A single serving of one popular frozen pepperoni pizza contains 2.5g salt (1,022mg sodium).
- One brand of chicken-vegetable soup has an amazing 5.9g salt (2,398mg sodium) per can.

Many foods now list salt or sodium on their labels, so choose low-salt types. To convert milligrams of sodium to grams of salt, divide by 1,000 and multiply by 2.5.

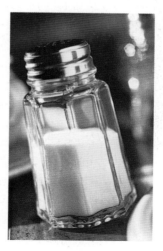

Compelling new evidence tells us that just about everyone could benefit from eating a little less salt.

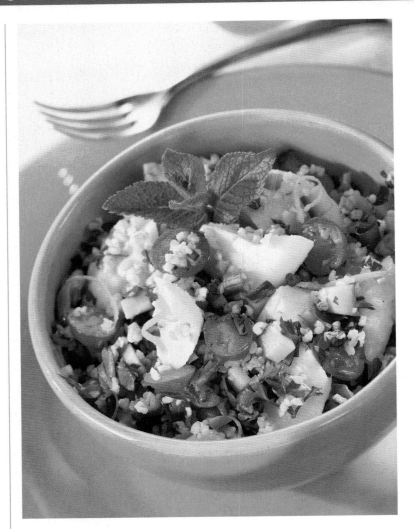

> If eating foods that contain protective substances is good for you, the thinking goes, taking a pill will be just as good. But is it?

Can't I just take a pill?

No sooner do researchers spot a substance in food that seems to fight disease than some clever entrepreneur begins to put it into pills or potions. Your local health-food store is sure to be packed with bottles containing all kinds of supplements, from vitamin E to multivitamins. But if eating foods that contain these protective substances is good for you, people say, surely taking a pill will be just as good. Or is it?

The evidence is still murky. People who fill up on vegetables and fruit loaded with the antioxidant beta carotene (such as carrots and mangos) have lower risk of heart disease than people who get little – but beta carotene pills have proved to have no benefit in several large studies. Worse still, some volunteers taking beta carotene had a higher incidence of lung cancer.

Another antioxidant that has researchers scratching their heads is vitamin E. In a report that made headlines in 1993, women who took vitamin E supplements daily cut their heart disease by 30 per cent. A study published three years later found that male heart patients who took a daily E capsule were half as likely to have a second heart attack.

Then came the Heart Outcomes Prevention Evaluation study, or HOPE – the largest and most carefully designed investigation of vitamin E ever undertaken in the USA. The volunteers, including 2,545 women and 6,996 men, were all at high risk of heart attacks, either because they had cardiovascular disease or risk factors for it, such as diabetes. Half began taking a dose of 400 international units daily – the equivalent of 268mg of vitamin E. The other half were given a placebo. Four and a half years into the study, the number of heart attacks, stroke and deaths in both groups was precisely the same. Vitamin E hadn't offered any protection at all.

No one can explain these contradictory results. Some experts think a daily capsule of vitamin E may be powerful enough to prevent the artery damage that leads to coronary artery disease but not potent enough to reverse the disease once it sets in. Others think taking the pills is a waste of money, given the latest findings. Several large studies currently under way should help to shed more light on the controversy. For now, most experts seem to agree that taking 540mg of vitamin E won't hurt you – and just might help to prevent heart problems down the road.

Multiple benefits

The diets of many people in the UK do fall short on some of the essential vitamins and minerals and, according to the British Nutrition Foundation, if you feel that your diet isn't meeting all your nutritional require-ments, for reasons you cannot control, then you may benefit from taking a multivitamin and mineral supplement.

▼ Key finding

In a 2001 study at Tufts University, researchers found that older people who took a multivitamin for eight weeks had higher levels of B vitamins in their blood and lower levels of homocysteine – a substance linked to heart disease risk.

If you decide to take a supplement, study its contents carefully and avoid any that offer high doses of single vitamins and minerals, which can be quite dangerous if you are not sure of what you are doing. If in doubt, consult a doctor, state registered dietitian or pharmacist. The best way to get all these nutrients is from foods, principally fruits, vegetables and whole grains, because they also provide fibre and other plant constituents that supplements cannot provide. Taking a multivitamin cannot replace a healthy diet.

Recipe for success

Good fat, bad fat. Complex carbohydrates, simple ones. Grams of salt and percentages of calories from fat. If you're feeling a little overwhelmed, relax. Healthy eating is really about making a wise choice each time you shop for groceries, sit down to order a meal, grab a snack or plan your next dinner. And you don't have to make all the right choices all at once. It's often easier to develop healthy eating habits meal by meal, day by day.

Your first step: pick one change you're prepared to make. Then formulate a plan for how you'll do it. Finally, keep track so you know how well you're doing. Let's say your goal is to eat an extra serving or two of fruit and vegetables a day. Decide how you'll make that happen – by adding berries or bananas to your cereal in the morning and an extra vegetable at dinner, for instance, or keeping baby carrots in the fridge as a snack. Try taking lunch to work, and including a piece of fresh fruit or a box of raisins, and putting lettuce and tomato on your sandwich. For the next couple of weeks, keep an informal food diary of what you eat at each meal. If you fall short of your goal now and then, don't give up. Just try to do better tomorrow.

Here are ten simple changes you can make that will help to protect your heart. This week, try to make two or three. Come back to the list after you've incorporated them and choose two more. Within a month, you will have gone most of the way toward adopting a heart-smart diet.

1 If you drink milk, switch to a lower-fat variety.

2 Have a bowl of wholemeal cereal for breakfast at least three times a week.

3 Have fruit instead of your usual dessert at least three times a week. (Try baked apples or a fresh fruit salad.)

4 Switch from white bread to wholemeal bread.

5 Instead of eating beef, choose fish, turkey, chicken or a very lean cut of pork most days of the week.

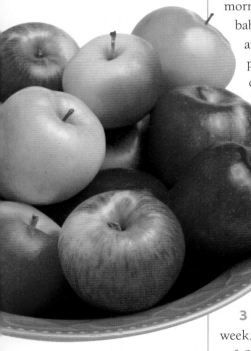

> It's often easier to develop healthy eating habits meal by meal, day by day.

6 Instead of ice cream, opt for sorbet or non-fat frozen yoghurt.

7 In place of potatoes or white rice, have wholemeal pasta or brown rice at least once a week. Why not experiment with grains you haven't tried before, such as bulghur wheat or barley?

8 Add one more vegetable to your dinner, either as a side dish or as part of the main meal. (Instead of pasta with meat sauce, for instance, opt for pasta primavera. Or try spinach lasagne.) Stock up with fresh vegetables and fill your freezer with frozen vegetables to help you to meet your goal.

9 Put an enticing bowl of fruit in a prominent place and help yourself when hunger hits.

10 Sauté foods in olive oil instead of butter or margarine.

Calories count

There is one last crucial component to heart-healthy eating: balancing calories. Being overweight or obese significantly increases the chances of developing heart disease – and almost 60 per cent of people in Britain now fall into these categories. This is because too many of us take in more calories than we burn up. If your body mass index, or BMI (see page 131), is in the healthy zone, you're doing fine and you don't need to worry. If your BMI is high, keeping an eye on the calories you take in is important. Chapter Seven takes a closer look at losing weight – and keeping it off.

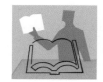

TERMS TO KNOW

ANTIOXIDANT A substance that neutralizes free radicals, unstable oxygen molecules that might otherwise damage healthy tissue

CARBOHYDRATE A chemical component of food that can take the form of sugars, starches or cellulose

CHOLESTEROL (DIETARY) A waxy substance found in the fatty tissue of animals (no plant foods contain cholesterol)

THE GLYCAEMIC INDEX (GI) is a term used to rank individual foods according to the effect they have on blood sugar levels, that is, how quickly they're digested.

INSOLUBLE FIBRE A type of fibre – found mainly in wholegrain cereal products – that helps to speed up the rate at which food passes through the digestive tract

MONOUNSATURATED FAT Heart-healthy fatty acids abundant in olive, rape seed and peanut oil

OMEGA-3 FATTY ACIDS A form of fat – found in oily fish, certain vegetables and seeds – that protects against heart disease

POLYUNSATURATED FAT Heart-healthy fatty acids abundant in corn, soya and safflower oils

SATURATED FAT A form of fat (found mainly in meat and dairy products) shown to increase blood cholesterol levels. 'Saturated' refers to the fact that every carbon atom is paired with a hydrogen atom

SOLUBLE FIBRE A form of fibre (found mainly in citrus fruits, apples, potatoes, dried peas and beans, and oatmeal) that can be dissolved by the digestive tract

TRANS FAT Artificially produced fat created by adding hydrogen to unsaturated fat molecules, making it solid at room temperature. Trans fats have been shown to raise cholesterol levels

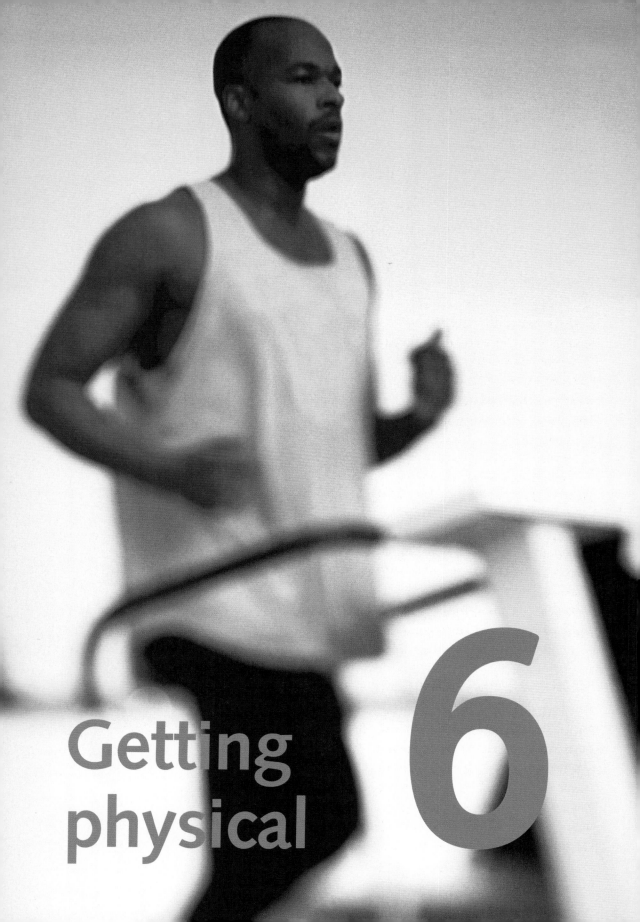

Getting physical

6

Figuratively speaking, your heart is the wellspring of your emotions. But literally, it's a muscular organ, and muscles need regular workouts. If the only time you work up a sweat is when you worry, it's high time to think about exercise. You don't have to take up running or even join a gym. Studies show that even moderately intense activities – such as brisk walking and ballroom dancing – will help you to live longer and stay healthier.

Exercise not only keeps your heart strong, making it less susceptible to damage, it also helps to maintain adequate blood flow to the heart and other parts of the body, keeping blood vessels in better shape. And that's just the beginning. When you give your muscles a workout, you make it easier for the cells throughout your body to process energy in the form of blood sugar, or glucose, which in turn helps to lower the risk of diabetes, which is a serious risk factor for heart disease.

Physical activity improves the ratio of good to bad cholesterol. Plus it reduces the risk of high blood pressure. People who are sedentary have a 30 per cent greater chance of developing hypertension than people who are moderately active. And of course, burning more calories by getting off the couch helps you to keep your weight under control, which is also crucial to the health of your heart.

Simply put, if a pill could provide as many benefits as exercise does, we'd all be clamouring to take it.

Public health enemy number one

We all know exercise is good for us, but 70 per cent of adults in the UK fail to meet government guidelines, which recommend at least 30 minutes of physical activity at least five times a week. One in three of us, according to the latest statistics, gets no exercise at all.

It's easy to understand why we've become a nation of couch potatoes. These days we almost have to go out of our way to be active. Labour-saving devices have taken over most tasks that used to be done manually, and our lives are easier as a result. But we have

If a pill could provide as many benefits as exercise does, we'd all be clamouring to take it.

Regular exercise...

1 Lowers blood pressure
2 Boosts HDL levels and reduces total cholesterol
3 Increases strength and stamina
4 Expands lung capacity
5 Boosts the immune system
6 Builds muscle
7 Burns fat
8 Reduces the risk of diabetes
9 Protects against colon cancer
10 Eases depression and anxiety
11 Helps to control your weight
12 Maintains strong bones
13 Allows you to stay active as you get older

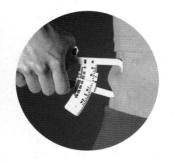

far fewer opportunities to get our hearts beating and our lungs working. People in the year 1900, going about their normal lives, burned almost 1,500 more calories every day than we do today.

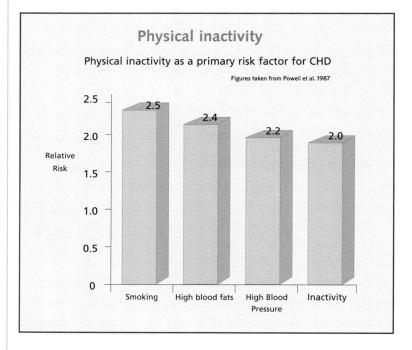

As you can see (above), nearly 20 years ago, researchers recognized that inactivity was a risk factor for heart disease. Recent research from the World Health Organization estimates that it causes around 3 per cent of all diseases in the developed world. Taking little or no physical exercise is hard on almost every part of the body. But it's especially hard on your heart. The British Regional Heart Study confirms that inactivity significantly increases your risk of heart disease. Our bodies, in other words, are meant to move.

Are you healthy enough to exercise?

Most people, even those with heart disease, can safely get out and exercise. However, don't overdo it. A study by scientists at Essex University found that infrequent, strenuous exercise poses a risk of heart attack.It's wise to check with your doctor before starting on a fitness programme, especially if any of the following apply to you.

- I've been diagnosed with coronary artery disease or another heart-related condition
- I sometimes feel pain in my chest when I do physical activities or when I'm under emotional stress

- I'm worried that other health problems I have may worsen with physical activity
- I'm over 69 years old

If any of these statements describe you, make an appointment to talk to your doctor before you begin a new exercise programme – particularly one that involves moderately strenuous activities.

Taking the right kind of exercise

Physical activities take two basic forms. The first, aerobic exercise, gets your heart beating faster and your lungs working harder. Examples include walking, jogging, dancing, swimming and cycling. You can tell an activity is aerobic if it leaves you feeling slightly or very winded.

The second, called resistance training or strength training, builds muscles, usually by making them lift, pull, push or otherwise move something heavy. The classic way to strength-train is with weights in a gym. But you can also do simple exercises using portable dumbbells or even your own body weight.

Both forms are important for overall health. Strength training is especially vital for maintaining what researchers call functional capacity – the ability to do what you like to do throughout most of your life, even when you are very old. Keeping your muscles strong helps you to keep your balance as you age and also to maintain a healthy weight, because muscle tissue burns more calories than fat does, even when you're sitting still. Having strong muscles, that are better able to take in energy in the form of blood sugar, lowers the risk of Type 2 diabetes, too.

But when it comes to your heart, aerobic exercise is more important. Researchers found that sedentary 60-year-old men who began an aerobic-exercise programme improved their

▼ Key finding

Adding moderate-intensity activity to your daily life increases the diameter of the arteries feeding the heart, which in turn boosts the amount of blood that reaches heart muscle. What's more, over time, new blood vessels begin to form, providing even more blood to the heart. Regular physical activity also increases the heart's efficiency. A study by researchers at the University of Leipzig in Germany found that exercise increased peak blood flow (the maximum amount of blood that can flow through arteries) by 200 per cent.

Tips for exercising safely

✔ Don't overdo it. Gradually ease yourself into a new activity programme

✔ Make sure you have a good pair of trainers and comfortable clothes

✔ If you walk or jog at dusk or at night, wear reflective clothing

✔ If you ride a bike, wear a helmet

✔ If you engage in sports that can involve falling, wear wrist and knee guards

✔ Drink about ¾ pint of water before and after you exercise

✔ Stretch before and after you exercise (see page 106 for some basic stretches)

✔ Warm up by starting off slowly and gradually increasing the intensity level

✔ If you're exercising vigorously, cool down at the end with 5 to 10 minutes of less vigorous activity

lungs' ability to take in and deliver oxygen by almost 12 per cent. The volunteers increased the amount of blood their hearts could pump by almost 10 per cent. Finally, their hearts became more efficient – this was measured by the percentage of blood leaving the heart during each heartbeat. All these improvements mean that more oxygen and nutrients reach all parts of the body, including the heart. And that has to be good news.

Tickle your fancy

Maybe you've put off exercising because you weren't sure how to begin. The first step is deciding what you'd like to do. Walk? Jog? Ride your bike? Swim? Join an aerobic-dance class? Take up a sport like tennis or squash? There is so much to choose from.

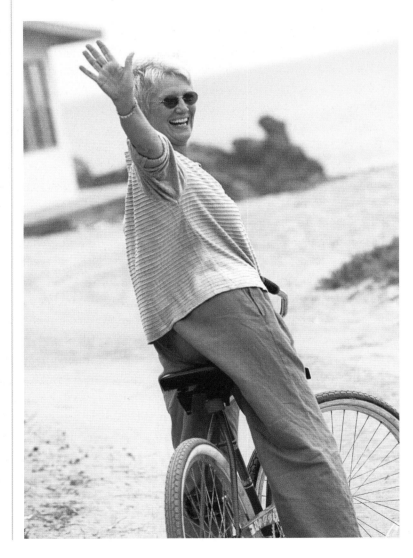

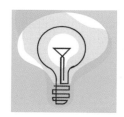

ASK THE EXPERT

How do I know if I'm exercising enough to help my heart?

Steven Blair Ph.D., director of research at The Cooper Aerobics Research Institute, in Dallas, Texas, and senior scientific editor of the 1996 Surgeon General's Report on Physical Activity and Health says:

The good news is that you don't have to do athletic-style training to get some benefits of exercise. All you have to do is about 30 minutes of at least moderate physical activity on most, preferably all, days of the week.

We're talking about sedentary adults – people who aren't doing much of anything at the moment. If you're already more active than that, stick with what you're doing. But if you're among the millions of people who aren't active, racking up 30 minutes, most days will go a long way towards protecting your heart.

What do we mean by moderate activity? The most common example is walking briskly at between three to four miles per hour. To check your pace, map out a mile course in your neighbourhood. Walk at your usual pace for a mile, checking your starting and stopping time. A brisk walk should take between 15 and 20 minutes. If yours takes longer, gradually increase the pace. Moderate-intensity exercise should leave you breathing harder and slightly warmer than usual.

The official recommendations also mention exercising for 30 minutes. There was a time, ten years ago, when exercise scientists thought you had to work out for a period of, say, 45 minutes to an hour to get heart benefits. Now we know

smaller segments of activity can add up to the same benefit. Three 10-minute walks have the same benefit as one 30-minute walk. How short can an activity segment be? Are 30 one-minute walks the same as one 30-minute walk? No one knows. No doubt there is a minimum duration. I suspect it may be around 5 or 6 minutes, but that's pure speculation. Still, if you've only got 5 minutes, it's better to spend it being active than sitting still. We sometimes encourage people to begin with 2-minute walks just to overcome the inertia that keeps many people sedentary.

Finally, we talk about exercising on most days of the week. I think it's wise to strive for 7 days a week, knowing that you're likely to miss a day here and there. If you accumulate 30 minutes of activity on at least 5 days a week, you're doing fine.

Will you get more benefit by pushing yourself harder? Sure. But our studies have shown that if you go from doing nothing to up to 30 minutes of activity most days of the week, you'll cut your risk of prematurely dying in half. Do more than that – an hour or more of strenuous activity – and you'll cut your risk by an additional 10 to 15 per cent. The biggest payoff comes from moving out of the sedentary group into the moderately active group.

A basic stretching routine

Stretching before exercise helps to prevent injury. Stretching also keeps you flexible, making it easier to do many physical activities. Here are four simple stretches to get you started. Hold each stretch for 10 to 20 seconds. Repeat four times on each side.

■ Calf stretch

Stand a few feet from a wall. Take a step forwards with your left foot. Keeping your right leg straight and both heels on the ground, lean forward. You'll feel your Achilles tendon, at the back of your foot, and your calf muscles stretch.

■ Hamstring stretch

Place the heel of your left leg on a low stool, step or anything you have to hand, such as an upturned bucket. Place your hands above your hips for support. Bend over very slowly, keeping your back straight and your shoulders square until you feel a stretch at the back of your leg.

■ Quadriceps stretch

Place your right hand on a chair or against a wall for balance. Grasp your left foot with your left hand and pull your foot gently toward your buttocks, keeping your standing leg slightly bent. You should feel the muscle at the front of your thigh stretch.

■ Lower-back stretch

Lie on your back with your knees bent. Using both hands, pull your left knee to your chest, pressing your lower back into the floor. You should feel the stretch in your buttocks and lower back.

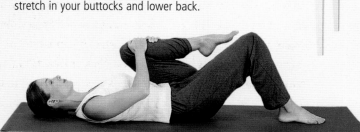

If you already know what to choose, that's great. If not, think about the kinds of activities for which you are most likely to have the time and motivation. Some people prefer regular workouts at a gym. Others prefer activities like bicycling, dancing, walking or organized sports. A third option is to incorporate exercise into your daily life, by walking instead of driving, taking the stairs instead of the lift or escalator, working in the garden or throwing a ball for the dog. Very active people usually combine several approaches.

What's right for you? Incorporating activities into your daily routine may be best if:

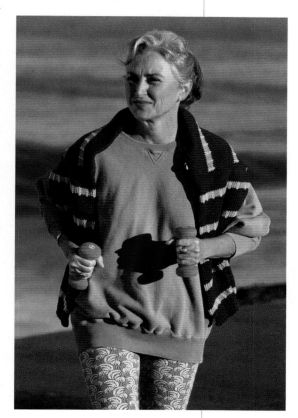

- You have trouble setting aside at least an hour three or four times a week to exercise
- You're uncomfortable with the way you look or embarrassed that you're out of shape
- You have a lot of chores around the house and garden to keep you busy
- You've just never been the gym-going type
- You enjoy walking

Joining a local gym or fitness centre may be the best option to choose if:

- You're motivated by having other people around
- You'd like to try classes in aerobic dance, yoga, Pilates or other activities
- You would benefit from the help of a personal trainer or fitness expert
- You have bought exercise equipment before and watched it gather dust as it sits in the corner

▼ Key finding

Moderate-intensity aerobic exercise could help you to avoid cold and flu bugs. According to a 1993 study, women who did a brisk 30-minute walk most days of the week reported half as many days with cold or flu symptoms than women who didn't walk. By increasing blood flow, researchers believe, exercise may boost the number of immune cells circulating through the bloodstream, enhancing the body's ability to detect and destroy invading viruses.

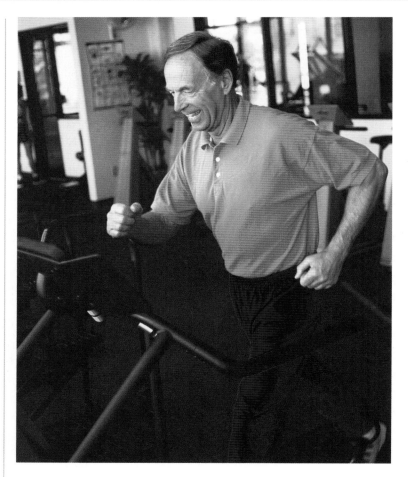

Joining the gym brigade

Twenty per cent of the UK population stay active by joining a gym, fitness centre or other fitness facility. There are many advantages to doing so. Most places have instructors who can show you how to use the equipment and create an appropriate workout plan. Many offer classes in aerobic dance, water aerobics, yoga, using an exercise bike, kick-boxing and other activities, as well as special programmes for older people. The simple act of joining a gym can represent a big step in your commitment to exercise.

Before you sign up, however, make sure the facility is right for you. Too many people join with all the best intentions, only to let their membership lapse when they end up not going. Consider these questions before you put down money.

- Is it conveniently located?
- Is the club well maintained and clean?
- Is the atmosphere comfortable?

- Does it offer everything you'd like (weight machines, pool, exercise classes, steam room, sauna)?
- Are the staff friendly and willing to help?
- Is the price right and would it suit you?

Once you've chosen a health club, make an appointment for an instructor to teach you how to use all the equipment – even before you've decided what kind of exercises you'd like to do. You may discover that you love using the cross-country ski machine or the elliptical trainer, but you won't know until you try them.

Gentle exercise

If you are not interested in joining a gym, it's no problem. You can get all the exercise you need by beefing up your everyday activities at home or around the neighbourhood.

The notion that lifestyle exercise can offer all the benefits of full-blown workouts is what US experts have called 'exercise lite'. When specialists first claimed that just 30 minutes of moderate-intensity activities could provide most of the benefits of more vigorous exercise, not everyone was convinced. So researchers at The Cooper Aerobics Research Institute in the USA decided to put the concept of exercise lite to the test. They recruited 235 sedentary men and

Moderate-intensity activities

1 Swimming
2 Cycling
3 Cycling on a stationary bicycle
4 Mowing the grass (with a push mower)
5 Raking
6 Dancing
7 Walking briskly
8 Mopping or scrubbing the floor
9 Golf (without a cart)
10 Tennis (doubles)
11 Volleyball
12 Rowing

Vigorous-intensity activities

1 Aerobic dancing
2 Climbing stairs or hills
3 Digging the garden
4 Tennis (singles)
5 Jogging
6 Hiking on hills
7 Downhill skiing
8 Cross-country skiing
9 Swimming laps

Keep an activity log

The great advantage to lifestyle exercise is that you can do it whenever you like and wherever you happen to be. The challenge is making sure small bouts of activity add up to at least 30 minutes a day. The simplest way is to keep an activity log in a small note-book. Each time you take a brisk walk or climb the stairs, jot down what you did and how much time you spent. Just before dinner, tally up your activities for the day. If you've fallen short of your 30 minutes, plan to take a brisk walk around the neighbourhood after you eat. Here's what an activity log might look like:

TIME	ACTIVITY	DURATION
7:00 – 7:15	Walked before breakfast	15 minutes
8:00 – 8:05	Climbed stairs at work	05 minutes
12:30 – 12:45	Walked during lunch	15 minutes
5:30 – 5:45	Raked leaves in garden	15 minutes
TOTAL		50 minutes

women. Half agreed to engage in a standard gym-based programme of exercises, with treadmills, stair-climbing machines, stationary bikes and all the rest. The others met once a week in small groups to talk about ways to incorporate physical activities into their daily lives, then followed up on their ideas.

At the end of two years, people in both groups had lowered their blood pressure by more than 3 points and lost the same amount of body fat (almost 2.5 per cent). And all the participants were burning exactly the same number of calories.

The results persuaded most experts worldwide that you really can create a heart-healthy exercise programme simply by looking for opportunities to get moving around the house, office and neighbourhood. There are only three rules.

Easy ways to add exercise

Opportunities abound to add exercise to your everyday life. Here are some examples.

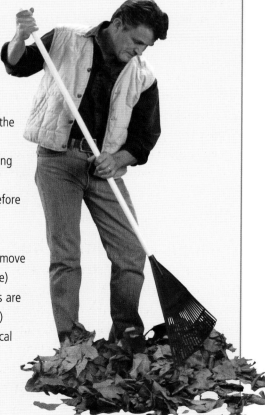

- Walking instead of driving to do errands or shopping within a quarter mile radius
- Trading in your ride-on lawnmower for a push model if your lawn isn't too big
- Raking leaves instead of using a leaf blower
- Getting off the bus one stop early and walking the rest of the way
- Parking at the far end of the car park and walking
- Taking stairs instead of lifts and escalators
- Walking a full circuit around shopping centre before you begin shopping
- Climbing stairs or walking during work breaks
- Volunteering for activities that keep you on the move (doing chores for elderly neighbours, for instance)
- Walking the dog (if you don't have one, chances are a neighbour's dog would love the extra exercise)
- Riding a bike instead of driving whenever practical (be sure to wear a helmet)
- Joining a local hiking or biking club
- Taking ballroom or line-dancing classes

1 The activities must be at least moderately intense – vigorous enough to leave you breathing harder and slightly warmer (adding more vigorous activities is fine, of course).

2 You'll need to accumulate at least 30 minutes of activity on most days of the week.

3 You'll need to keep track of how much activity you do.

Count your steps

If your activity of choice is walking or jogging, you can also use a clever gadget called a pedometer, or step counter, a small device that fastens to your belt or waistband and records each step you take. Pedometers work by way of a small pendulum that swings each time you step. The basic idea is not new : measuring steps can be traced back to the Romans, and Leonardo da Vinci experimented with pedometers. Thomas Jefferson is said to have introduced them to America. Then, 40 years ago, the '10,000 Steps a day' programme was introduced in Japan.

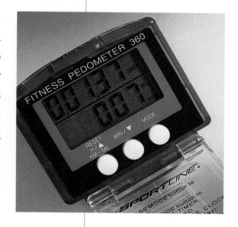

In 2004, pedometers were back in the spotlight after several studies found that walking 10,000 steps a day – the equivalent of about 5 miles – was an effective way to combat widespread obesity. It reduces body fat, lowers body mass, tones legs and slims waists.

Put on your pedometer in the morning and see how many steps you have taken by the end of it. Take the average for a week and try to build that up by 10 per cent a week.

Step counters are available at sports shops, and cost from £7.50 to £20. The Walking the Way to Health initiative offers them by mail order; contact www.whi.org.uk or call 01242 553 258.

Walking your way to better health

In October 2000, the Countryside Agency and the British Heart Foundation launched the Walking the Way to Health projects which aims to improve the health and fitness of more than a million people, especially those who do little exercise and live in areas of poor health, by getting them walking in their own communities. Hundreds of walking schemes have started up, in England and Wales, organized by local volunteers. They guide short walks, with information about the places on the way. The Scottish initiative is called Paths to Health and their website is www.pathsforall.org.uk

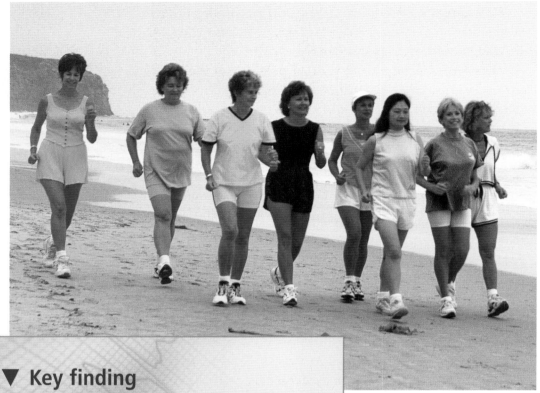

▼ Key finding

In 2004, proof of Britain's reluctance to exercise was revealed by the National Office of Statistics, who interviewed 14,800 people in England, Scotland and Wales about their sport and leisure activities. It found that only 59 per cent had undertaken at least one physical activity and only 35 per cent had walked at least two miles in the previous four weeks.

It's no wonder that walking has become one of Britain's favourite forms of exercise. You can do it almost anywhere. You don't need to join anything. In fact, the only equipment you need is a pair of comfy shoes.

Getting started

If you haven't done much walking, start slowly and gradually increase the time you spend and the distance you cover. Here's a month-long programme to start you off on the right foot. For safety's sake, always let someone know where you'll be walking and when you plan to be back.

Week one Set a goal of walking at least 15 minutes a day, at least five days this week. Walk at whatever pace feels comfortable. Don't worry about the distance you walk.

Week two Increase the time you walk to at least 20 minutes. Push yourself a little more – you should have to breathe a little harder and feel slightly warmer.

Week three Aim for a total of 30 minutes a day at least five days this week. Get into the habit of walking first thing in the morning and just before or after dinner.

Week four Walk 30 minutes at least four days this week. Try to keep your pace brisk. On another day set aside time for a 45-minute walk. To keep it interesting, plan to walk somewhere pleasant, like a local park or along a riverside.

Once you've built up to walking 30 minutes a day, you can be flexible with your walking routine. Take longer walks when you have the time. On busy days, break your walks into 5 or 10-minute outings and try to accumulate two or three of them.

Sensible walking

A few simple tips can help you to get the most out of walking and protect yourself against injury.

Start slowly By gradually picking up your pace over the first minute or two, you'll get your heart and muscles primed before you hit your stride.

Walk tall Keep your shoulders back and relaxed and your stomach tucked in to protect your lower back. Keep your chin up to prevent strain on your neck. Your eyes should be focused ahead, not on the ground.

Find your stride Walk steadily, letting your arms swing freely by your sides. The best rhythm and stride for you is the one that

Choosing a walking shoe

You don't really need special walking shoes – all you need is a pair of comfortable shoes. But if you are buying new shoes what really matters is comfort. If it feels good, chances are it provides enough cushion and support. When you're shopping for shoes:

■ **Try on both shoes** Left and right feet are often slightly different in size. Find a pair that fits your larger foot.

■ **Wear the socks** you plan to exercise in. That way you'll make sure the fit is right.

■ **Allow a little extra room** Your feet swell a little through the day, so buy trainers with a thumb's-width worth of extra space between your longest toe and the end of the shoe. Make sure the overall fit is snug. If your heel slips or your foot can roll from side to side, the shoes are too loose and may cause blisters or even injury.

feels most comfortable and natural. If your strides are too long your head will bob up and down with each step.

Find soft surfaces Concrete and tarmac are hard on knees and hips. A better bet is soft dirt roads, trails or running tracks.

Listen to your body If you feel pain in your joints or muscle stiffness, ease up a bit. If the pain continues, consult your doctor.

Add slowly As you gain confidence and fitness, increase the speed or duration of your walks. To avoid strains, add no more than 10 per cent a week to the time you spend on each walk.

Stretch After walking gently for five minutes, stop and stretch. Then do it again at the end of your walk to keep you supple and to avoid stiffness. See page 106 for four basic stretching exercises.

REAL PEOPLE, REAL WISDOM

Running in her father's memory

Helen Streeter, aged 30, had always led an active life. While she was at university she played for the ladies' football team, attended exercise classes and swam.

After university, Helen took on a physically demanding job and often felt very tired after work. So she would sit in front of the TV and just couldn't find the energy to exercise. But then, on New Year's Eve 2003, her father suffered a fatal heart attack.

'It was completely unexpected,' she says. 'But I knew straight away that I wanted to do something positive, instead of sinking into depression. So I decided to run for a charity that funds heart research.'

Although she wasn't as fit as she used to be, Helen decided to train for the Great North Run, a half-marathon from Newcastle to South Shields, which takes place every September.

She asked an old university friend, Gemma, who lives close by, if she would also take part in this event. Gemma agreed and they started training in February 2004 for the September event. 'It was tough at first', she laughs. 'But it's much more fun with a friend – she's faster than I am, so when I hurt, she reminded me why we were running. It was a great way to keep motivated.'

When the day of the race arrived, Helen was among some 49,000 competitors. She noticed that many of the runners were older – in their sixties and seventies, but as fast or faster than she was and quite undaunted by the difficult terrain. 'It was very tough', she says. 'I didn't remember the course being that hilly.'

Helen finished the race in 2hr 39min – very close to her target time – and raised a total of £850 for the National Heart Research Fund. 'I knew it was going to be hard but then I just thought of my dad and why I was doing this and the run became easier.' Helen is now quite determined to keep up her running. 'It's good for vascular health,' she says, 'and it's a great way of keeping physically and mentally fit.'

A good stretch for walkers is toe circles. To do these, stand on one foot, point the toes of your other foot and trace circles in the air, both clockwise and counterclockwise. Repeat with the other foot.

Looking at home exercise equipment

If you have some extra space and cash, you can set up your very own exercise room at home. A US study suggests it can be well worth the money. The scientists enlisted 148 overweight women and divided them into three groups. Women in the first group walked 40 minutes at a shot, five days a week. Those in the second group walked 10 minutes at a time, for a total of 40 minutes. The third group also did 10-minute walk segments but with a crucial difference: The research team lent them treadmills to use at home. Eighteen months later, the treadmill group had lost over 16lb (7kg). The women in the other two groups had lost between 8lb and 13lb (3.5kg and 5.7kg). These results suggest that people with a treadmill end up getting more exercise.

But you can also put together a simple home fitness centre with an exercise mat (for sit-ups and stretching exercises), a small set of dumbbells (for strengthening exercises) and a skipping rope and exercise video (for aerobic exercise). If you find you enjoy working out at home, you could treat yourself to a stair machine or treadmill.

Before you buy anything, however, be sure you'll use it. Too many of us spend money on home exercise equipment only to see it gather dust. Before you spend your money:

1 Make sure there's a comfortable place in your house If working out means going into a damp basement or dusty garage to use your exercise equipment, the chances are you'll find a dozen reasons not to do it.

▼ Key finding

Making any lasting change takes some effort and commitment. Along the way, it's important to reward yourself for a job well done. Think of something fun you can do for yourself when you meet your weekly exercise goal – a dinner at your favourite restaurant, for instance, or new workout clothes. Researchers found that people who used rewards as a way to motivate themselves were almost twice as likely to stay active than those who didn't.

continued on page 118

Easy at-home muscle toning

These six simple exercises require nothing more than a little bit of room and a carpet or exercise mat. You can do them at home or when you're travelling. If you're exercising for the first time in a while, go easy – especially if you have back problems. Do as many repetitions as you can comfortably manage. A 20-minute session three times a week is all you'll need for good overall muscle toning.

■ Sit-ups

These help to tighten the abdominal muscles. Lie on your back with your knees bent. Keep the small of your back pressed against the floor. With your hands behind your head, fingers touching and elbows pointing out, curl your upper body about a quarter of the way toward your knees. Use your abdominal muscles to accomplish this; do not pull on your neck. Hold for 2 seconds, then lower yourself back to the floor.

■ Cobra (press-ups)

This exercise is great for strengthening your abdominal muscles and lower back. Lie face down with your hands near your shoulders, palms against the floor. Exhale as you start to straighten your arms to raise your upper body off the floor; keep your hips and lower body relaxed and on the floor. Stop when you feel a stretch in your lower back or waist. Hold for 2 seconds, then lower yourself to the original position.

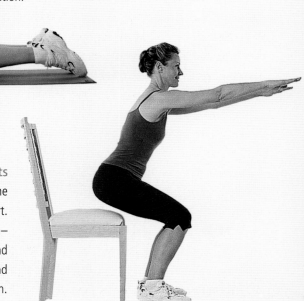

■ Squats

These target the quadriceps muscles at the front of the thighs. Stand with your legs about shoulder-width apart. Slowly lower yourself as if you were sitting on a chair – and just about as far – keeping your back straight and leading with your buttocks. Don't let your knees extend past your toes. Then raise yourself up again.

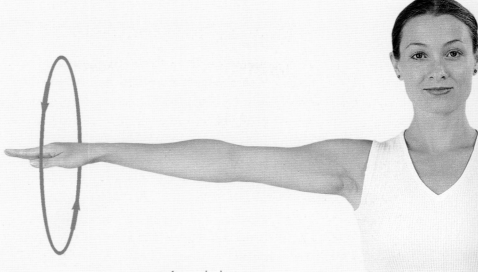

■ Arm circles

These will tone your arms, shoulders and chest muscles. Extend both your arms outwards, as if you were preparing to fly. Then make small, slow circles with them, about as big around as a dinner plate. When your arms begin to tire, reverse the direction of your circles.

■ Knee hug

This is a great exercise for lower-back muscles. Lie on your back with your knees bent and your feet flat on the floor. Exhale as you use your abdominal muscles and hips to pull your knees towards your chest. With your arms behind your knees, palms on elbows, pull your knees closer to your chest. Hold for 2-3 seconds, then release your legs, lowering your feet slowly to the floor. Repeat. To increase the stretch, raise your chin to your knees as you hug your knees.

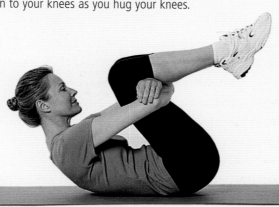

2 Find out about hiring Search the internet for companies that hire out stair-climbing machines, rowing machines, treadmills and other exercise equipment. Hiring is a good way to try out different machines and see much you might use them, before you buy.

3 Evaluate carefully before you buy Visit several stores before you buy. Compare the features different models offer, and be sure to try a piece of equipment to see how it feels. Then, you might want to search eBay to see if anyone is selling the equipment you like at a bargain price.

4 Ask about a maintenance agreement Some equipment, such as treadmills and stair-climbing machines, need frequent adjustment and repair. Having a maintenance agreement could help to guarantee that when a piece of equipment breaks down, you get it fixed and back on track fast.

Your plan of action

Whether you've decided to enroll at a gym, join a sports team or add more physical activity to your everyday life, it's important to write up a plan of action. After all, it's one thing to tell yourself that you're going to become more physically active; it's another actually to do it. And the best way to make any change in your life, experts say, is to have a plan. Your action plan should include:

- A list of the kinds of physical activities you intend to do
- A schedule for exactly when and how long you will engage in these activities
- Your activity starting date
- How you plan to keep track of the amount of activity you do

Once you've drawn up your action plan, mark your activities on your calendar for the next four weeks. Write down everything you intend to do: workouts at the gym, 15-minute walks during lunch hour, jogging with the dog. Then tell at least one family member and one friend about your resolution to become more active. Get in the habit of checking your calendar in the morning and again in the evening. Keep track of the activities that you completed and those you didn't get to.

During the coming month, don't worry if you miss a day or two. It doesn't mean your resolution has crumbled. It only means you've missed a day or two. Look back at your calendar, check to see what you've scheduled for tomorrow, and get back on track.

FAST FACT
A Finnish study recently found that fit men and women were two to five times less likely to die of coronary artery disease than people who were physically unfit.

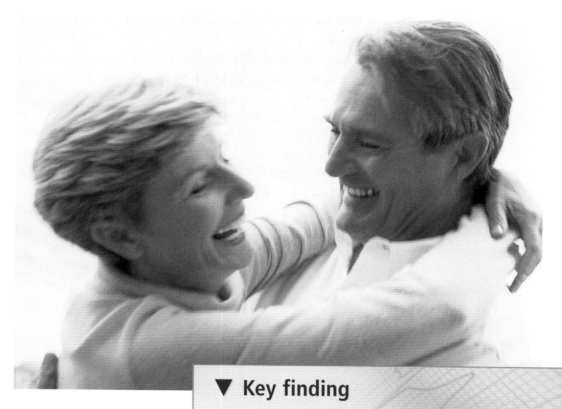

▼ Key finding

Older adults who take part in exercise programmes are not only healthier but also happier, according to research carried out in the USA. Scientists studied 60 women who were older than 60 who were living either independently or in communities where some care was provided. The women who were the most physically active rated their quality of life higher than those who were inactive, no matter where they lived.

Charting your progress

Once you have started your programme of heart healthy activity, you'll want to know you're making progress. Of course, by simply getting up and doing something when otherwise you would have been sitting around, you've made headway. Here are some of the benefits you may reap.

More stamina Exercise scientists measure fitness by how long someone can walk or run on a treadmill. Fancy equipment can also measure how much oxygen the lungs can take in during strenuous exercise. But the simplest gauge is whether you can do activities like brisk walking or jogging for longer than before or whether you're able to increase the intensity of your activities – riding a bike up steeper hills, for instance, or walking a mile in 18 minutes instead of 20. If so, you're increasing your fitness level.

Hot topic:

What's the best way to measure intensity?

Back in the days when exercise gurus thought you had to do strenuous activities to reap the health benefits of exercise, the usual way to gauge exercise intensity was measuring heart rate. The goal was to work out hard enough to get your heart rate into a certain range – your target heart rate (see below, left). But some experts aren't sure that heart rate is the right yardstick, or even a safe one, especially if you're aged over 50. Medical conditions and certain prescription medications can affect how fast your heart beats. Beta-blockers, for instance, tend to keep your heart rate slower. Arrhythmias, or irregular heart beats, can also affect heart rate.

Using a target heart rate as your guide is controversial for another reason. The latest evidence suggests that you don't need to get your heart rate high to gain benefits. A better measure, many experts say, is the Borg Perceived Exertion Scale, which scores how difficult a particular activity feels to the person doing it (see below, right).

In the end, the best method depends on how fit you are now and your exercise goal. If you're already active and want to increase your level of fitness, the target heart rate approach will give you the most accurate idea of how hard you're working your heart and lungs (provided you don't have a medical condition or take drugs that affect your heart rate). If you're just beginning an exercise programme and your goal is to be active enough to protect your heart, the Borg scale is your best choice.

THE TARGET HEART RATE

Your heart rate is an indication of how hard you're working. The more intense your workout, the faster your heart has to beat in order to provide enough oxygenated blood to muscles. Target heart rate – the pulse you're aiming for during vigorous exercise – varies with age. See the numbers below. If you're taking high blood pressure medication, your target heart rate might be lower; check with your doctor.

AGE	TARGET HEART RATE
30	95–142
40	90–135
50	86–127
60	80–120
70	75–113
80	70–105

THE BORG PERCEIVED EXERTION SCALE

Use this scale to describe how much you feel you're exerting yourself – from not at all to very, very hard. A score of 13 to 15, the 'somewhat hard' to 'hard' category, should put you roughly at your target heart rate. If your score falls below 10, try to push yourself a little harder. If your perceived exertion is above 17, ease back a bit to make sure you're not overdoing it.

6 – No exertion at all
7 – Very, very light
8
9 – Very light
10
11 – Light
12
13 – Somewhat hard
14
15 – Hard
16
17 – Very hard
18
19 – Very, very hard
20 – Maximum
    exertion

Lower blood pressure Many people with hypertension who become more active see a drop in their blood-pressure readings over time. One study showed that aerobic exercise reduces resting blood pressure in people who have hypertension by an average of 11 points off the top number and 9 points off the bottom one. For many people, that's enough to bring the numbers down into the safety zone.

Improved cholesterol ratio Exercise often lowers LDL (the 'bad' cholesterol) slightly, but its biggest benefit is in increasing HDL, or 'good' cholesterol. Volunteers in a study who began walking or jogging 9 miles a week saw their HDL levels climb 13 per cent.

Lower resting heart rate Regular exercise makes your heart and lungs work more efficiently. That often means your heart will beat more slowly as you stick with your new activity regimen. A lower resting heart rate is a sign of cardiovascular health.

Weight loss What most people hope for when they begin an exercise programme is to lose a few pounds – and if you're over-weight, you probably will. But be patient: losing weight through exercise is a slow process, because when you exercise, you exchange fat for muscle. And muscle tissue weighs more than fat because it is denser. So the numbers on the scale may not budge right away. But you will be improving your body composition – and looking better in the mirror. And because muscle burns more calories than fat, increasing your muscle mass also boosts your metabolism. So over time, getting fit will help you to maintain a healthier weight.

More self-confidence Becoming active is likely to boost your confidence level, especially if you've been sedentary. You will look better and feel better. And if you master an activity or two that you couldn't do before – aerobic dance or strength-training exercises, for instance – you'll enjoy a sense of accomplishment.

Overcoming obstacles

If you're like most people, your carefully laid plans of becoming more active will come up against obstacles that seem to set you back – like a rocky period at work or a spell of foul weather that foils your daily walk. Sickness, holidays, even just a bad mood, can

Not seeing the progress you hoped for? Don't be discouraged. Not everyone benefits in the same way from exercise. Some people lower their blood pressure dramatically; others see barely a drop. Some lose a lot of weight; others lose very little. Whether or not you are making measurable changes, you are strengthening your heart and lowering your risk of a heart attack. In a study of 21,925 men, researchers discovered that volunteers who were obese but physically fit – measured by performance on a treadmill test – were less likely to die from heart disease than slim men who were unfit.

make it hard to keep to your resolution. But for every obstacle, there's a way around it. For example:

When the weather turns frightful There are plenty of ways to exercise indoors. You can walk around a shopping centre or at the local gym if there's a track. Or rent an exercise video.

What's it worth?

Here are the number of calories you can expect to burn doing various activities. Of course, these are only averages. For more activities, log onto www.caloriecontrol.org/exercalc.html

ACTIVITY	ESTIMATED CALORIES BURNED PER MINUTE OF ACTIVITY			
	120LB/54KG PERSON	160LB/72KG PERSON	200LB/90KG PERSON	240LB/108KG PERSON
Walking, 30-minute mile	2.4	3.2	4	4.8
Bowling	2.9	3.8	4.8	5.7
Dancing (waltz, fox-trot, samba)	2.9	3.8	4.8	5.7
Mopping, vacuuming	3.4	4.5	5.6	6.1
Cycling, 10 miles an hour	3.9	5.1	6.4	7.6
Water aerobics	3.9	5.1	6.4	7.6
Weeding or digging in the garden	4.3	5.7	7.2	7.9
Aerobic dance, low impact	4.8	6.4	8.0	9.5
Walking, 15-minute mile	4.8	6.4	8.0	9.5
Playing tennis (doubles)	5.8	7.7	9.6	11.4
Horseback riding (trot)	6.3	8.3	10.4	12.4
Swimming laps (moderate effort)	6.7	8.9	11.1	13.4

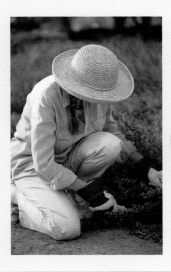

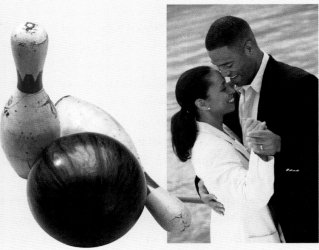

When work gets hectic Remember that exercise can be a terrific antidote to stress. Taking just a 10-minute break for a brisk walk will clear your head and give you new energy to tackle problems. Or you might choose to get up a little earlier and exercise before work. That way, no matter what the day brings, your workout won't get squeezed out of your schedule.

If the people around you get in the way Friends and family should encourage you to become more active. But that isn't always the case. Some people close to you may feel threatened by your new resolve to exercise. Some may even try to sabotage your efforts. If that's the case, sit down and talk about why becoming more active is so important to you. If appropriate, encourage family or friends to join you.

When the holidays hit Make physical activity a priority by scheduling it on your calendar. If you have family visiting, explain to them beforehand that you'll be taking time out to exercise. You can also incorporate exercise into family activities, by ice skating, hiking or walking on the beach together.

If you're feeling down A fit of the blues can make it hard to find the energy to do anything. That's the time to remind yourself that physical exertion can lift your spirits by triggering the release of mood-elevating hormones called endorphins. Some studies show it can even ease symptoms of full-fledged depression. If you just can't rally your spirits for your normal workout, at least go for a walk in a place you enjoy. You may find that getting up and doing something makes it easier to return to your exercise routine.

Moving forward

After the first month, see how well your action plan is working. If you've kept an activity log, look it over. Use the quiz on page 125 to evaluate your progress.

If you're satisfied with what you did the first month, think about pushing yourself a little harder. The more active you are, after all, the healthier you'll be. If your goal is to lose weight, beefing up your exercise routine is especially important. The longer you engage in physical activities, and the more intense the activity, the more calories you burn.

When the second month is over, re-evaluate your action plan one more time. If you're feeling a little bored with what you're doing, try a few new activities. You may find that there all kinds of opportunities to get moving, in your local community.

Join the club

Many communities offer an array of clubs and classes to help to get you into the exercise groove. Look for:

1 Cycling clubs
2 Golf clubs
3 Walking clubs
4 Running clubs
5 Nature rambles
6 Badminton clubs
7 Squash clubs
8 Rowing and canoeing clubs
9 Water-aerobics classes
10 Tennis leagues
11 In-line skating clubs
12 Ski clubs
13 Ballroom and other dancing classes
14 Environmental activities, such as beach and riverside clean-ups

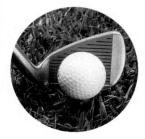

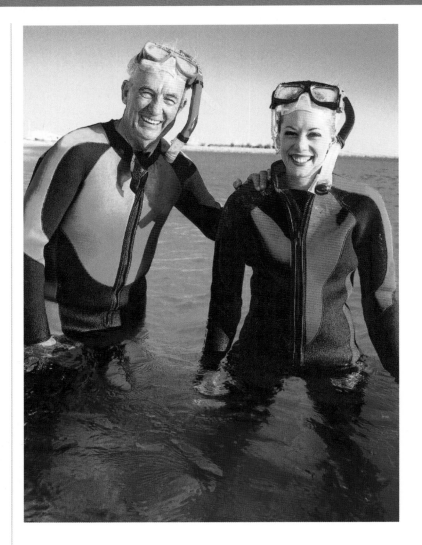

Remember, too, that no one is perfect. You will probably go through periods when you aren't as active as you'd like to be. Now and then, you may fall off the exercise bandwagon entirely. The worst thing you can do is decide that you've failed and abandon your plan. If you falter along the way, get up, dust yourself off and start again. Over time, physical activity may well become one of the best parts of your life – your chance to do something good for your heart, body and spirit. Sign up for a cycling or walking holiday, and it could take you to exciting new places and you'll meet like-minded people.

TROUBLESHOOTING TIP

If you feel the need for some help in planning your exercise programme, why not try one of the many get-fit initiatives available in the UK? BUPA has teamed up with GetFit to give you a safe, easy way to plan an exercise programme and build or maintain your fitness. Simply log on to GetFit. This is not a free programme, however. More details from www.bupa.co.uk

How am I doing?

1 During the last month I met my activity goals:
- Every day
- Most days
- Half the time
- Less than half the time
- Seldom or not at all

2 The biggest obstacle for me was:
- Not enough time
- Feeling down
- Trouble at home
- Getting bored with one activity
- Stress at work
- Other _____

3 What I like best about being active is:
- The chance to take a break from work to get up and move
- Spending time with other people
- Getting out in the neighbourhood
- Feeling that I'm doing something good for myself
- Gaining confidence
- Other _____

4 What I dislike about being active is:
- Having to force myself to do something I don't feel like doing
- Taking time out from a busy day
- Working hard and not seeing the results I wanted
- Having to exercise on my own
- Feeling self-conscious about how I look
- Other _____

5 The most powerful motivator for me is:
- Setting a goal and sticking with it
- Putting exercise times on the calendar
- Exercising with someone else
- Rewarding myself with something fun
- Other _____

6 I would come closer to meeting my goals if:
- I had someone to exercise with
- I had more time
- I enjoyed what I was doing more
- My friends were more encouraging
- My schedule was less hectic
- Other _____

Not meeting your goals? Look back at your answers to fine-tune your action plan.

Item 2: Think of creative ways around your obstacles. If you're bored with walking, add a different activity, like bike riding or swimming.

Item 3: Write down other benefits you're getting. Stick the list on the refrigerator. When you're tempted to skip your scheduled activity for the day, look at it.

Item 4: Think of ways to take the bother out of exercising. If you're self-conscious about the way you look while exercising, rent exercise videos or consider buying a treadmill for your home. Or treat yourself to smart new workout clothes. If you dislike working out alone, sign up for an exercise class.

Item 5: Find ways to get even more out of the things that work best for you. If setting goals really helps, make yours as specific as possible.

Item 6: Turn at least one item on your wish list into reality. If you wish you had more time, identify an activity that you're willing to give up. If you don't enjoy what you're doing, try out other activities until you find one you do like.

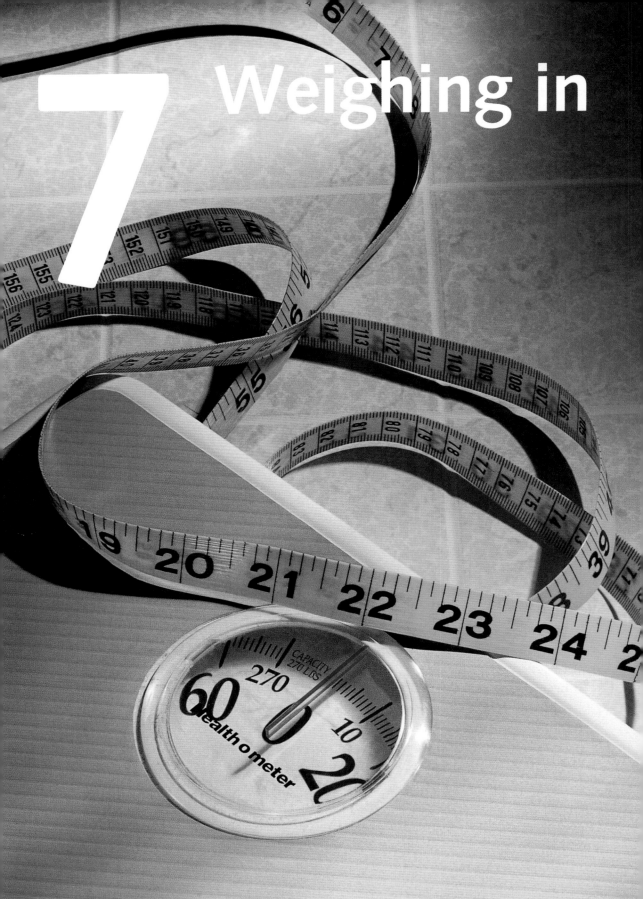

7 Weighing in

The health of your heart may not be your main reason for wanting to lose weight, but perhaps it should be. Shedding even a few excess pounds can lower your cholesterol and blood pressure and reduce your risk of Type 2 diabetes – significantly cutting your chances of having a heart attack or a stroke. Of course, weight loss will also help you to look better, feel better and have more energy.

If you're hoping to lose a little weight – or even a lot – you're not alone. Almost two in five women in the UK and one in six men say they are on a diet most of the time. Losing weight isn't easy, but it's not impossible. There are thousands of success stories from people who've done it. You can do it, too. There is no secret formula and you don't have to banish a long list of foods from your diet.

If you've begun to adopt some sensible eating habits and to add more physical activity to your daily routine, you're already on the way to losing weight. To advance, you'll need to keep a keen eye on the calories you consume and to concentrate on burning more calories by being more active.With all the high-protein, reduced-sugar, fat-fighting diet plans around, it's easy to forget that calories and energy expended are what matter when trying to lose weight.

A calorie is a tiny measure of energy, so the calories in food are a measure of the energy they contain – the fuel you need in order to function. (In fact, food values or the energy your body burns to maintain all its systems and be active are generally measured in thousands of calories – kilocalories or kcals, though still loosely known as calories. A gram of fat contains 9 kilocalories; carbohydrates and proteins have 4 kilocalories per gram.) Calorie intake determines how much you weigh. Consider these facts:

1. If you consume more calories than you burn, your body will store the excess as fat, and you'll gain weight.
2. If you consume fewer calories than you burn, your body will have to burn fat for energy, and you'll lose weight.
3. If you strike a balance between calories in and calories out, you'll maintain a stable weight.

That's all there is to it – the 'secret' of body weight, in three very simple equations. They are so obvious that you probably already know them. All you have to do is apply them.

> **With all the high-protein, reduced-sugar, fat-fighting diets available, it's easy to forget that calories are what matter when you're trying to lose weight.**

Why you?

Chances are you've wondered why you have to struggle with your weight when other people you know can eat all they want and stay slim. Certain factors do make it easier for some people to put on the pounds – and a little harder to take them off. In other words, gaining or losing weight is more than just a matter of willpower. Five factors may play a role.

1 Genes Being overweight or obese runs in families. If both parents have weight problems, it is likely that seven out of ten of their children will, too. If only one parent is overweight, the odds drop to four in ten. If the weight of both parents' is normal, their children have only a one in ten chance of a weight problem. One method that researchers use to examine the powerful role that genes play is by looking at identical twins.

Rate your readiness

How motivated are you to lose weight? To find out, answer the following questions. Then add up the scores beside the answers you've circled.

How do you feel about the prospect of losing weight?
- Very enthusiastic 4
- Moderately enthusiastic 3
- Willing 2
- Discouraged 1

How do you rate your chances of reaching your weight-loss goal?
- Excellent 4
- Very good 3
- Good 2
- Poor 1

How important do you think losing weight is for your heart?
- Very important 4
- Important 3
- Fairly important 2
- Not very important 1

How would you describe your attitude to restricting the amount of food you eat?
- Very willing 4
- Willing 3
- Resigned 2
- Reluctant 1

How easy is it for you to stop eating, even if there is still food on your plate?
- Very easy 4
- Easy 3
- Difficult 2
- Almost impossible 1

How willing are you to give up doing something you like in order to have more time for physical activity?
- Very willing 4
- Willing 3
- Resigned 2
- Reluctant 1

Studies have shown that twins raised apart are very likely to weigh exactly the same when they grow up, no matter how or where they were raised or who raised them.

But genes aren't destiny. Having overweight parents doesn't mean you'll be fat no matter what you do – it just means you'll probably have to work a little harder to maintain a healthy weight.

2 Glands 'It's a glandular problem', people often used to say about being overweight. The gland in question is the thyroid, which is located in your neck, just above your voice box. The thyroid controls your metabolism, which affects how many calories you burn while you're at rest.

Having an overactive thyroid (hyperthyroidism) means you burn more calories than normal. An underactive thyroid (hypo-thyroidism) causes you to burn fewer than normal.

Which of these statements do you think describes your understanding of what it takes to lose weight and keep it off?
- I know what it takes 4
- I'm pretty sure I know what it takes . . 3
- I'm confused by conflicting advice and diet plans. 2
- I don't know what will work for me . . 1

If your favourite food is in the house, how easy is it for you to resist eating it?
- Easy 4
- A struggle, but I can do it 3
- Difficult 2
- Almost impossible. 1

Do you have people close to you who will support you in your weight-loss goal?
- Yes, many. 4
- A few. 3
- One 2
- No 1

Which of the following statements best describes you?
- If I set my mind on doing something, I can do it. 4
- I'm pretty good at meeting my goals . 3
- Even when my intentions are good, things seem to get in the way 2
- I get easily discouraged 1

A score of 34–40 means you're ready and willing to begin a weight-loss programme. A score of 25–33 means you're almost ready.

A score of 10–24 suggests that you should spend some time and effort mentally preparing yourself before you begin.

If your score falls into one of the last two categories, write down your reasons for wanting to lose weight. Then add two more potential benefits. Write down three of the biggest obstacles you face – and at least one strategy to help you to overcome each obstacle. Finally, think about occasions when you've changed something in your life. What helped you to succeed? How can you use a similar strategy to lose weight?

Some weight problems do stem from an underactive thyroid – but not many. Fewer than 5 per cent of overweight or obese people can really blame this gland. If you think you might fall into that category, talk to your doctor. (Other symptoms of underactive thyroid include lethargy, intolerance to cold temperatures, aching muscles, constipation and fluid retention.) If blood tests reveal an underactive thyroid, medication can set it right. But don't assume it will be a magic bullet. You'll still have to do what everyone does: balance calories in and calories out.

3 Metabolism Some people burn more calories than others, even when they're sleeping or doing nothing at all. There are many reasons for this. Muscle tissue requires more energy to maintain than fat does, so if you're muscular, your resting metabolic rate, or RMR, may be a little higher than someone who has little muscle and a lot of fat. (That's one reason exercises that build muscle help you to stay slim.) Some people inherit what researchers have dubbed a 'thrifty gene' – an inherited tendency to conserve energy greedily. As a result, they have a lower RMR. Sophisticated tests can measure your RMR. But there's not much point to having such a test done, since the weight-loss prescription is still the same: consume fewer calories and burn up more.

4 Fat cells Fat is stored in specific cells that make up adipose, or fatty, tissue. Some people have larger-than-normal fat cells; others have more fat cells than normal. An obese person can have around 260 billion fat cells; a slim person may have only 25 billion.

If you've been overweight since childhood, there's a good chance that you may have more fat cells than the average person. That doesn't mean you can't shed some of those pounds, however. No one has ever shown that having too many fat cells makes it harder to lose weight.

5 Personality traits Most people tend to overeat when they are feeling sad, lonely or anxious. Many overweight people say they often eat – and overeat – when they're emotionally distressed.

Psychological factors like this probably play a role in determining why some people struggle with their weight and

▼ Key finding

You don't have to lose a lot of weight in order to take the burden off your heart. A 1995 study found that when overweight people lost as little as 8lb (3.5kg), their blood pressure, LDL cholesterol and triglycerides went down. At the same time, their HDL cholesterol levels rose, improving the ratio of 'good' to 'bad' cholesterol – exactly the kind of changes that dramatically lower the risk of a heart attack.

Body mass index (BMI)

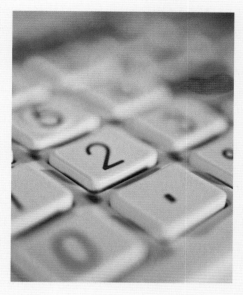

Most people use only scales to determine if their weight is healthy. But this isn't the best measure because it doesn't take into account

height or body type. A much more accurate measure is body mass index, or BMI. Log on to www.medicdirect.co.uk for help in calculating your BMI. Or you could work it out using either of these formulae:

1 **Divide your weight in pounds by your height in inches squared. Then multiply the total by 703.**
Example: 145 ÷ (64 x 64) x 703 = 24.8

2 **Divide your weight in kilograms by your height in metres, squared.**
Example: 65 ÷ (1.62 x 1.62) = 24.8

The World Health Organization classify a BMI of between 18.5 and 24.9 as healthy and a BMI of between 25 and 29.9 as overweight. A score of 30 or above indicates obesity.

others don't. By learning to recognize what real hunger feels like (see page 142) and distinguishing it from food cravings, you can go a long way towards eating not to comfort yourself but to satisfy an empty stomach.

Though some or all of these factors may be part of the reason you're overweight, the main culprit is consuming more calories than you burn. If you keep that firmly in mind, it will be much easier to lose weight and keep it off.

The way to lose weight

There are plenty of weight-loss plans, but finding the one for you is not easy. The bookshops are full of them, each competing for your attention. With millions of frustrated dieters looking for answers, there is plenty of money to be made in offering the secret of successful weight loss. A lot of diet plans are based on nothing more than gimmicks and some of them are actually dangerous,

Proof Positive

Diets don't work, the gloomy headlines report. Most people who lose weight gain it back again – and often a few extra pounds as well. Is losing weight a lost cause?

'Absolutely not,' says dietitian Paula Hunt. 'It's crash diets that are the problem. They produce a fast initial weight loss, but your body needs the chance to adjust – which is what happens when weight loss is slow, at a rate of, say, a pound or two a week.'

One such programme has been going for more than 40 years. The WeightWatchers ethos has four simple principles: a healthy balanced diet; an increase in physical activity; a group environment; and behavioural support from trained leaders who have followed the programme themselves.

Members choose a food plan that is easy to stick to – no food groups are cut out, so they do not feel deprived and end up binge-eating or yo-yo dieting. The food plan is based on a points programme, where members eat a certain number of points a day, from any type of food. The new WeightWatchers programme is based on two years' research with 1,000 successful members who have lost weight and kept it off for more than 18 months. Some of the small changes that helped them to lose weight were identified as:

- Making wise food choices.
- Getting support.
- Managing your thoughts.
- Learning from experience.
- Planning ahead.
- Managing your feelings.
- Measuring and recording.

Research has shown that losing weight in a group environment is more successful than trying to do it alone. Attending the meetings, and knowing that you're among people who know what you're going through is a great motivator. To find a WeightWatchers group near you, call 08457 123000 or visit their website at www.weightwatchers.co.uk

especially if you're at risk of heart disease. For instance, although there is some evidence that high-protein diets do cause people to lose weight at first, some protein-rich foods also tend to be loaded with artery-clogging saturated fat that is dangerous to many people.

Look closely at the most popular diet plans, and you'll discover that nearly all of them offer roughly the same thing: a way to help people to cut back on calories. One diet, for instance, contains a long list of foods to avoid, including carrots, sweetcorn, peas, sweet potatoes, bananas, raisins, fruit juices, as well as most grains and breads. Ban those foods from your menu and you're almost certain to shed pounds, regardless of the complicated theory behind the diet. There's a better way to lose weight, however, and it doesn't involve banishing whole categories of foods from your plate. All it takes is making small adjustments to what you eat, how much you eat and the amount of exercise you get. Over time, those adjustments can add up to a real difference on the scales – and your risk of heart attack. There is a four-week programme, beginning on page 134, to get you started.

How low should you go?

How much weight can you reasonably expect to lose? If you're overweight or obese, most experts say it's sensible to begin by setting a goal of losing about 10 per cent of your current weight. If you hit that mark and still have a way to go to reach your ideal healthy weight, you can always set another target. Whenever you

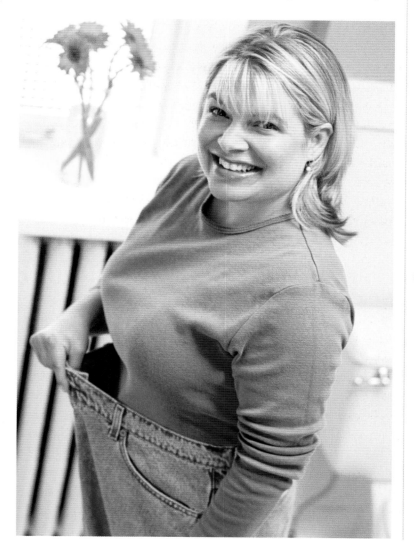

Most popular diet plans offer roughly the same thing: a way to help people to cut back on calories.

need encouragement, remind yourself that studies show that losing just 4 per cent of body weight can dramatically lower elevated blood pressure and cholesterol levels – which reduces your risk of heart disease and other chronic illnesses.

How fast should you aim to shed those pounds? Researchers say it's both reasonable and safe to lose up to a pound or two (up to a kilo) a week. To do that, you'll need to consume fewer calories and burn more calories through exercise.

Week one: keeping a food and activity diary

To shift your calorie balance towards weight loss, it helps to know how many calories you now consume and roughly how many you burn. The food and activity diary on page 137 is designed to help you to do that. A good idea is to make a month's worth of photocopies of the diary and place them in a ring binder file.

During the first week, concentrate on making a note of everything you eat and exactly how much time you spend doing physical

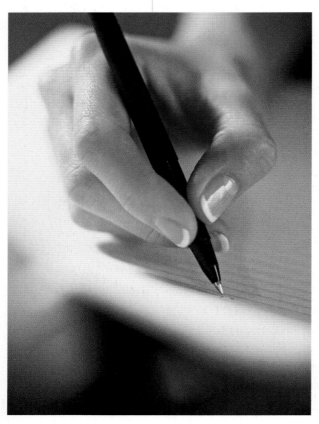

activities. Tracking your food intake will make you more conscious of the food choices you make and the calories they involve. If you find that you are cutting back on portion sizes or refusing that rich dessert because you're suddenly aware of how many calories it contains, that's fine. But don't start dieting in earnest just yet.

Packaged-food labels state precise calorie counts per serving. But for fresh foods you'll need to buy a calorie counter – a book that lists thousands of foods and the calories they contain. Many bookstores have them. Many good recipe books now give nutrient analyses for each portion.

It is a good idea to buy a small notebook that you can carry around to jot down what and how much you eat during the day. Then, at the end of the day, fill in your diary, including

Diet vs exercise

To lose weight and keep it off you'll need to exercise and watch your calorie intake. Many people find it helps to start by concentrating on one or the other approach. Each has its advantages. If you're in a hurry to lose pounds, for instance, dieting should be your first plan of attack since it offers quicker results – and it's easier for most people to cut back on the calories they consume than to burn an equivalent number through physical activity.

If you're more concerned with how you look in the mirror than with numbers on the scale, exercise may be the way to go, since it tones your muscles while burning fat. Read the following statements and tick 'Yes' or 'No' to determine where to focus your efforts.

- I prepare most of my meals at home. Yes ■ No ■

- My main goal is to look and feel more toned. Yes ■ No ■

- I'd like to use my scales to plot how my weight loss progresses. Yes ■ No ■

- I'm under a lot of stress and it sometimes gets me down. Yes ■ No ■

- I'm good at planning ahead, especially when it comes to where and what I'll be eating for breakfast, lunch and dinner. Yes ■ No ■

- When I sit down to a meal, I have difficulty saying no to foods I love. Yes ■ No ■

- My schedule is hectic, which makes it hard for me to set aside time for myself every day. Yes ■ No ■

- I enjoyed sports and other physical activities when I was younger. Yes ■ No ■

- I have back problems or other physical conditions that make it hard for me to take regular exercise or be very active. Yes ■ No ■

- I'm not very good at keeping track of things like calories or grams of fat. Yes ■ No ■

- I've tried dieting before, and it just hasn't worked for me. Yes ■ No ■

- The main reason I want to lose weight is to lower my risk of heart disease. Yes ■ No ■

- I've become so heavy that I'm embarrassed to be seen even just out walking. Yes ■ No ■

- I eat a lot more fast food and junk food than I should. Yes ■ No ■

- I'm so out of shape that I just don't have the energy and strength to pursue new interests or do things that I'd really like to do. Yes ■ No ■

Scoring: Add up the number of answers that fall in pink boxes and the number in blue boxes. If nine or more of your answers are in pink boxes, you're best suited to a programme that emphasizes exercise. If nine or more are blue, a programme that focuses on diet may work for you. If your answers are evenly divided between blues and pinks, start off with a programme that combines diet and exercise.

the number of calories you've consumed and the number you've expended doing physical activities (see the chart on page 122 in Chapter 6 to help you estimate this or, for a more complete list of activities and how many calories they burn, try logging onto www.caloriecontrol.org/exercalc.html).

At the end of the week, look back over your diary. You may be surprised at how many calories you expend. Or you may be startled to see how many you consume.

The point of this first week is to gauge what your calorie intake and activity level are now. Take a few minutes to calculate the average number of calories you consume each day (add up the seven daily totals and divide by seven). Do the same to calculate the average number of calories you expend through physical activity.

SAMPLE FOOD AND ACTIVITY DIARY

Use the form (right) to keep track of the calories you consume and those you expend through exercise. Here's an example of what one day's entries might look like.

TIME OF DAY	FOOD	SERVING SIZE	CALORIES CONSUMED	ACTIVITY	TIME SPENT	CALORIES EXPENDED
6:30 AM	• Orange juice • All Bran • Skimmed milk • Coffee (black)	small glass 30g/1oz 150ml/5floz mug	55 81 48 0			
7:15–7:30				Brisk walk	15 minutes	105
10:00	• Doughnut	1 small	242			
12:30–1:30 PM	• Tuna sandwich with lettuce and tomato • Diet cola	1 330ml can	400 0			
3:30	• Apple	1	47			
6:00–6:30				Stationary cycling	30 minutes	300
7:30	• Salmon steak • Pasta with tomato sauce • Green beans • Wholemeal roll with butter • Wine • Fruit sorbet	100g/3½oz 150g/5oz 3tbsp 1 small glass 1 scoop	180 200 19 205 99 58			
TOTAL			1,634			405

FOOD AND ACTIVITY DIARY

TIME OF DAY	FOOD	SERVING SIZE	CALORIES CONSUMED	ACTIVITY	TIME SPENT	CALORIES EXPENDED

Week two: easing back on calories

During the second week, your goal is to begin to reduce the calories you consume. One strategy is simply to eat less. But it's also important to make sure that you don't go hungry. Otherwise, you won't last long on your weight-loss plan.

By making sensible food choices, you can sometimes eat more and still take in fewer calories. For instance, if you resist a slice of apple pie, which contain 200 calories, and choose a baked apple with 111 calories instead, you will still be enjoying a satisfying dessert for far fewer calories. A serving of potato salad contains 390 calories but if you opt for steamed vegetables with only 48 calories, you can have a plateful.

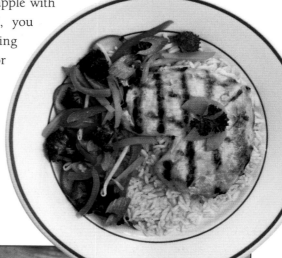

| Hot topic: | **Extreme dieting** |

Just as some diets promote high protein consumption, others trumpet the virtues of a very low-fat regimen. There are diets that focus on carbohydrates and diets built around certain foods. Do any of these approaches help people lose weight faster or more easily?

Some foods do seem to satisfy hunger on fewer calories than others. Protein, for instance, has been shown to trigger satiety, or the sense of fullness, faster than fat. And high-fibre foods, such as vegetables and whole grains, fill you up faster than foods with little or no fibre. But there's very little evidence that diets very high in this or very low in that offer any special benefits when it comes to losing weight and keeping it off. Consider a study conducted by

researchers at Geneva University Hospital in Switzerland. One group of volunteers was given a diet made up of 32 per cent protein, 15 per cent carbohydrates and 53 per cent fat.

The second group ate a diet composed of 29 per cent protein, 45 per cent carbohydrates and 26 per cent fat. Even on these very different diets – one with only 15 per cent and the other with 45 per cent of calories from carbohydrates – all volunteers lost the same amount of weight and the same amount of body fat.

What really matters, many experts now say, is how many calories you consume, not where they come from. The best diet for that is one that strikes a reasonable balance – and one you can live with for the rest of your life.

How many calories a day should you have, ideally? The answer depends partly on how many calories you burn, of course. For women, a weight-loss diet should contain roughly 1,200 calories. For men (because they typically burn more calories), a reasonable goal is about 1,500 calories. Studies have shown that people who successfully lose weight and keep it off consume around 1,400 calories a day. Many begin by cutting back to about 1,200, then gradually increasing their intake as they reach their goal.

Look back at your diary to see the average number of calories you consumed each day. If you averaged more than 500 calories over the goal of 1,200 (for women) or 1,500 (for men), you may want to ease yourself down to the new target. For this week, set a goal halfway between what you consumed last week and the target goal. If you're within 500 calories, you're close enough to set 1,200 or 1,500 calories a day as your goal.

Filling up on less

Unless you're eating packaged food, it's not easy to know how many calories an item contains. You don't need to know exactly, but a few simple rules can help to guide you toward the foods more likely to fill you up on fewer calories.

1 Choose foods high in fibre A bowl of porridge is more likely to satisfy your hunger than a bowl of sugar-coated corn-flakes. A three-bean salad will fill you up faster on fewer calories than a similar-sized portion of pasta salad. That's because foods loaded with fibre satisfy a hearty appetite on fewer calories than low-fibre foods do.

One reason is that fibre tends to absorb water, so it expands in your stomach. High-fibre foods are also more filling because it takes your stomach longer to break them down into useable energy than almost any other food; as a result you feel full for longer because your stomach is full for longer.

Some fibres (found in bran, whole grains, vegetables and the skins of fruits) can't be digested at all. These fibres fill you up without adding any calories to your diet and so are an important part of any attempt to lose weight.

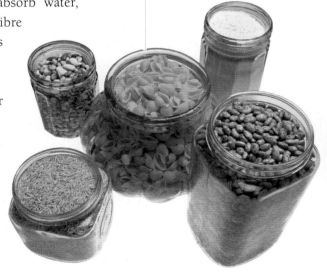

2 Cut down on fats Fatty food isn't the only culprit when it comes to body fat. You can put on pounds eating carbohydrates and protein, too. However, there's a good reason to hold back on fats, especially saturated fats. As mentioned earlier, fat contains 9 calories compared to only 4 calories per gram of carbohydrates – more than twice as many. In addition fats are much more easily digested; your body burns about 25 per cent more calories digesting complex carbohydrates such as fruits and vegetables than fat. (Simple carbohydrates, such as sugars, are more quickly absorbed.) Start by looking for ways to eliminate saturated fats. Enjoy bread without covering it with butter. Order fish or chicken that's roasted or grilled, not fried. Help yourself to low-fat yoghurt instead of ice cream. To lose weight, you may also need to reduce your intake of heart healthy unsaturated fats as well. Instead of pouring on salad dressing, for instance, drizzle just enough to moisten the leaves and add flavour, or choose a fat-free dressing.

3 Favour complex over simple carbohydrates All carbohydrates are eventually broken down into glucose, but not all of them are created equal. The simple kind are made up of only one or two sugar molecules. Complex carbohydrates consist of long chains of linked sugars. These take much longer for the body to break down. As a result, blood-sugar levels climb more slowly and remain elevated for longer, heading off hunger. Instead of a sugary soft drink, reach for tomato juice, for instance. And opt for wholemeal instead of white bread.

4 Choose nutrient-dense foods Especially when you're cutting back on calories, it's important to ensure you get all the nutrients you need. That's why you should choose nutritious foods, rather than empty calories. A 25g (1oz) serving of dry-roasted peanuts contains 147 calories – about the same as a similar-size serving of potato crisps. But nuts are loaded with vitamin E, protein and heart healthy unsaturated fats – unlike crisps, which offer little in the way of healthy nutrition. Surprisingly, studies have shown that people who often eat nuts typically weigh less than people who avoid nuts. Even a small handful can be more satisfying than a stack of fat-free crackers. Choose unsalted nuts as a high salt intake is associated with high blood pressure.

5 Increase the volume Foods that take up a lot of space (think of popcorn vs a small piece of cheese) tend to satisfy hunger on fewer calories, according to Pennsylvania State University

> Surprisingly, studies have shown that people who often eat nuts typically weigh less than people who avoid nuts.

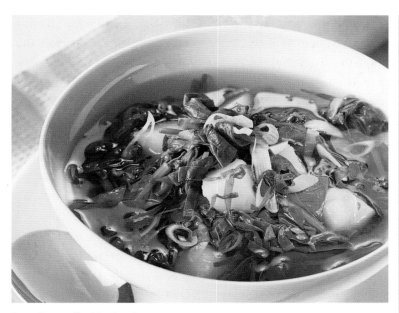

Start dinner off with a bowl
of broth-based soup, and you'll
consume fewer calories in
total by the end of the meal.

Ten high-volume, low-calorie foods

1 Plain microwaved popcorn
2 Broth-based soups
3 Whole-grain cereal
4 Most fruits (except dried fruits)
5 Green vegetables
6 Low-fat yoghurt
7 Puffed-wheat cereal
8 Unsweetened tea
9 Tomatoes
10 Vegetable juice

nutrition researcher Barbara Rolls Ph.D., co-author of *Volumetrics*. In a 2000 study Dr Rolls found that men who ate whipped-up yoghurt milk- shakes in the morning ate less at lunch. The more air the milkshakes contained (and thus the greater their volume), the fuller the men felt afterwards. Dr Rolls has also shown that people feel full for longer after having a bowl of chicken and rice soup than after eating a chicken and rice casserole with exactly the same number of calories. The reason is that broth is mostly water, so it fills you up on very few calories.

Join the slow food movement

Not long ago, food lovers from around the world founded a new movement called Slow Food. Its aim was to counter the trend toward fast-food eating habits and encourage people to cherish the joys of good food by finding better tasting (and much healthier) alternatives to, say, burgers and chips – and taking the time to savour every mouthful.

Consider your own eating habits. It is very likely that you often grab something to eat and bolt it down without paying attention to how it tastes. All those calories – and you didn't take the time to enjoy them! This week, try to slow down and pay attention whenever you sit down to eat. Follow these few simple tips, and you're likely to eat less and enjoy it a lot more.

Drop everything else When it's time to eat, do just that. Don't have a meal on a tray while you're watching TV, or eat while you're driving, or do a crossword puzzle while gobbling down lunch. Sit down somewhere and give the meal or snack all your attention. People who eat while distracted by other activities typically overeat because they're not paying enough attention to know when they've had enough to be satisfied.

Stick to a timetable Whenever possible, have your meals at roughly the same hour every day. Some people find it even helps to schedule meals, the way they schedule meetings. By setting aside a particular time to eat, you'll give the meal the priority it deserves.

Put your knife and fork down between bites If you eat too quickly, you won't give your body the chance to register the calories you've consumed and to send your brain the message that you've had enough. One reason many of us eat too much, experts say, is that we eat too fast. It can take up to 20 minutes for your body to signal that you're full. If you put down your cutlery between bites you'll slow down the rate at which you eat and, quite probably, eat less.

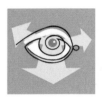

LOOKING AHEAD
A prickly weight-loss solution

For thousands of years the Hoodia cactus, a native plant of South Africa, has been used by bushmen to stave off hunger during long hunting trips. Someday it could provide a boon to anyone seeking to lose weight. Scientists have isolated one of the plant's active chemical compounds, dubbed P57, thought to suppress appetite. The compound is now in the early stages of testing on humans.

Serve smaller portions At home, where you can control the amount you have on your plate, give yourself half the amount you would normally have (you can always have more if you are still hungry). After you've finished the first serving, take 5 minutes to relax before taking more. Before you do, think about whether you're really hungry. If you are, have another helping. If not, leave the table.

If you're not enjoying it, don't eat it When you're cutting back on calories, every bite counts. If you are not enjoying what you're eating, put it aside.

Never feel you have to clean your plate Instead of beginning a meal with the goal of finishing what's in front of you, begin with the goal of satisfying your hunger. As soon as you no longer feel hungry, put down your cutlery and stop eating. This applies most particularly in restaurants, where very large helpings are served.

Five tasty ways
to cut calories

Low-fat foods don't have to be bland. Talented chefs use several tricks to give food big flavour without adding unnecessary fat or calories. Here's how you can, too.

■ **Choose high-flavour ingredients** A fresh parmesan cheese costs a little more than finely grated parmesan in a shaker tub, but it also has a stronger flavour, so you'll need less to make a dish tasty. Instead of adding minced beef to spaghetti sauce, add a highly seasoned hard Italian sausage, such as chorizo, and dice a few pieces to create a spicy meal with less fat. Use reconstituted dried mushrooms in savoury dishes for a concentrated taste sensation. Or try splashing a little sherry or wine into sauces to boost their flavour without adding fat.

■ **Sprinkle on herbs** Butter isn't the only ingredient that gives a rich flavour. Experiment with herbs and other seasonings to please your taste buds. Add oregano, thyme and a bay leaf to a soup made with lentils and vegetables for a delicious and nutritious dish. Dried fruits, such as apricots, prunes or raisins, and a scattering of Middle Eastern spices like cumin or cardamom turn rice into an exotic dish. Rosemary is perfect with chicken dishes, potatoes and roasted vegetables. If fresh herbs are hard to find or too expensive, used dried herbs, or consider starting a window-box herb garden with a few of your favourites.

■ **Chop it up** By slicing ingredients or dicing them into small pieces, you'll release more of their flavour and increase the volume of the dish, making a medium-size portion seem bigger. (Another trick to make a modest meal seem larger: serve it on smaller plates.)

■ **Less is more** In traditional Asian and Mediterranean cultures, meat was hard to come by, so home cooks learned simple ways to make a little go a long way. Try combining a small amount of chorizo sausage with beans in a pasta sauce or tossing in plenty of vegetables and tofu along with a bit of chicken for an easy stir-fry.

■ **Be colourful** What chefs love best about fruits and vegetables are the colours they bring to a meal. Nutritionists celebrate them because they're low in calories and fat and also high in fibre which makes a meal feel more filling. You can brighten up the appearance and the taste of almost any dish – from tuna casserole to a breakfast omelette – by adding chopped broccoli, sweetcorn, asparagus or diced tomatoes.

Eat only when you're hungry

When energy stores dip low, the body sends out physical signals in the form of hunger pangs to remind us to take in calories. Unfortunately, most people rarely wait that long. They eat food not because they're physically hungry but because of all kinds of psychological cues. If you're used to having a tub of popcorn every time you go to the cinema, for instance, you'll crave one as soon as you buy your ticket – even if you've just had dinner

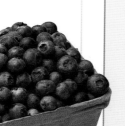

A LOW-CAL MENU THAT WON'T STARVE YOU

How well can you eat and still stay under 1,400 calories a day? Let's face it, you won't be snacking on Danish pastries or indulging in a chocolate decadence for dessert. But you can enjoy three satisfying meals – with a couple of healthy snacks thrown in. Here's what a typical under-1,400-calorie menu looks like.

FOOD	SERVING SIZE	CALORIES
BREAKFAST		
All Bran (small bowl)	30g/1oz	81
Skimmed milk	150ml/5fl oz	48
Strawberries or blueberries	75g (2¾oz	20
Orange juice (small glass)	150ml/5fl oz	55
MID-MORNING SNACK		
Apple or pear	1 medium	51
LUNCH		
Chicken salad sandwich on wholemeal bread		350
Orange	1 medium	56
Bottle of water		0
SNACK		
Tomato juice	200ml/7fl oz	28
Roasted unsalted cashews	25g/1oz	150
DINNER		
Salmon steak (grilled)	1 small	180
Green beans	75g (2¾oz)	19
Boiled new potatoes	3	113
Mixed green salad with 1 tbsp of French dressing		75
Low-fat yoghurt	1 pot	117
Strawberries	75g (2¾oz)	20
TOTAL:		**1363**

If your goal is 1,200 calories a day, replace the dressing on the salad with a fat-free dressing and eat 5 dried apricots instead of the cashew nuts.

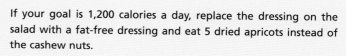

'A lot of the people we see in our weight-loss programmes have never really learned to identify true hunger', says John Foreyt Ph.D., a weight-loss expert at Baylor College of Medicine in Houston, Texas. 'They misconstrue all kinds of other feelings as hunger – which means they often eat even when they aren't really physically hungry.' According to Dr Foreyt, we often eat when we're feeling stressed, lonely, bored or anxious.

Can you resist all those psychological cues and eat only when you're hungry? Absolutely, the experts say. However, first it helps to know what real hunger feels like – and the simplest way to do that is to skip a meal. When you are truly hungry, your stomach feels empty. You'll probably begin to feel distracted and preoccupied with the thought of eating.

What about those times you find yourself ravenous for chocolate or something salty? Actually, you're not genuinely hungry; you're only experiencing a psychological craving. When that happens, change what you're doing or where you are. Get up and take a quick walk round the block or do a couple of chores around the house. Often the craving will pass. Then you can wait until your body needs food before you raid the refrigerator.

Reaching your calories goal

At the end of week two, look back over your daily calorie consumption. If you met your goal, congratulate yourself. If not, don't be discouraged. You're making progress simply by becoming aware of what you eat and how many calories your meals contain. If you need to bring your calorie consumption down further:

- Review your food diary and identify at least three items you can live without. Eliminate foods low in nutrients and high in calories, like sweets or salty snacks.
- Identify at least three items you can eat less of by cutting back on portion size.
- Identify at least one food that can be replaced with something lower in calories. If your breakfast cereal contains more than 200 calories per serving, for instance, try a puffed wheat or a rice cereal, which fills a bowl with under 100 calories.

TROUBLESHOOTING TIP

When dining out, avoid the temptation to fill up on bread before your order arrives. If you can see that the portions are very large, ask for a small helping or tell the waiter that you don't want the chips or roast potatoes. Another trick: drink plenty of water. One reason that people tend to overeat in restaurants is to keep their hands and mouths busy. Sipping water is a sensible, no-calorie solution.

- Plan to eat at least one additional serving of vegetables a day this coming week, either steamed or very lightly sautéed in olive or rape seed oil. The fibre in vegetables will help to fill you up on the fewest possible calories, so you'll be more able to resist higher-fat, higher-calorie foods.

Week three: burning more calories

Now that you are beginning to control the calories you consume, it's time to turn your attention to the other side of the calorie balance equation: the calories you burn. Most studies show that the only reliable way to lose weight and keep it off is to diet and exercise, because by burning additional calories through physical activity, you can increase the number of calories you consume and still maintain a healthy weight. The result is being able to enjoy a satisfying amount of food.

Any physical activity will do. The exercise of choice among most dieters is walking – it's easy to get started and you don't need any special equipment other than a good pair of shoes. On average, successful weight-losers burn about 400 calories a day through exercise. For a 10½ stone (68kg) person, that means walking four to five miles at a brisk pace – roughly an hour's worth of walking – every day. You might be able to achieve it by abandoning the bus or car while you diet and walking to work or to the shops. If you can't afford the time, find an activity that burns more.

Look back at your food and activity diary for last week. Work out how many calories you burned each day. Then calculate the average by adding the daily totals and dividing by seven. Subtract that number from 400 to see how many additional calories you need to burn in order to reach the goal of 400 a day.

This week, seek any opportunity, however brief, to burn up calories. Take the stairs instead of the escalator or the lift. Even skipping or jogging in place for 4 minutes instead of sitting on the couch during the TV commercials will help.

Of course, it is quite obvious that the more vigorous the activity – and the longer you engage in it – the more calories you will burn. Use your food and activity diary to keep track of your calories in and calories out.

TROUBLESHOOTING TIP

If you find you are not shedding pounds as fast as you'd like, don't get discouraged. For some people, losing weight takes longer than it does for others. Even if the numbers on the scale haven't moved, as long as you're adding more exercise to your life, you're losing fat and replacing it with muscle. And that will make it easier to keep the pounds off once you do begin losing weight.

WAYS TO BURN 400 CALORIES

A sure way to burn 400 calories is by taking a long, brisk walk. Turn this into a daily habit and your work is done. On the other hand, you don't have to expend those calories all at once. Here are some different suggestions, based on a 10½ stone (68kg) person.

ACTIVITY	TIME	CALORIES
Brisk walking	65 minutes	400
	TOTAL	400
Brisk walking	30 minutes	180
Sweeping patio or drive	10 minutes	50
Bowling	45 minutes	150
Vacuuming	5 minutes	20
	TOTAL	400
Brisk walking	30 minutes	180
Low-impact aerobic dance	30 minutes	180
Climbing stairs	5 minutes	40
	TOTAL	400
Vacuuming	15 minutes	60
Raking leaves	10 minutes	100
Swimming easy laps	30 minutes	240
	TOTAL	400

Week four: staying on track

Look over your diary for the past week and add up your calorie totals (both calories consumed and calories expended) to see how close you came to meeting your goal. If you didn't quite make it, identify some of the obstacles that hindered you. Then think of a few strategies to get around them. For example:

Can't find the time for exercise? Think of ways to relax in an active way. Arrange to meet friends for a walk instead of talking on the phone. Buy a stationary bike so that you can pedal while you watch your favourite TV programme.

Having trouble keeping track of what you eat? Buy a small notebook that you can fit into your pocket and take it everywhere you go.

Are restaurant meals your downfall? Identify a few local restaurants that offer delicious low-calorie choices and reward them with your business.

Overwhelmed by trying to change so many things? Most people have trouble tackling too many lifestyle changes at once. It helps to start with just one change; once you have that one under control, you can move on to another.

FAST FACT

When people diet without exercising, they lose not only fat but also muscle which, in turn, slows down their metabolism, causing them to burn fewer calories.

Remember that everyone has good days and bad days – periods when they stick to their goals and periods when they struggle. But people who succeed over the long term have one thing in common: they remain firmly committed to their goal even in the face of occasional setbacks. The more determined you are to lose weight, the more likely you are to succeed.

REAL PEOPLE, REAL WISDOM

Secrets of a successful loser

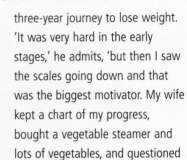

'They used to call me fatty,' says Gary Watson, 37, who lives in Portsmouth. 'All my clothes were XXL, but I thought nothing of it.' It had started in his mid-twenties when he learned to drive. 'I used the car for silly things like getting the paper and milk from the local shop, telling myself I needed the experience on the road.' Gary was training to be a chef, and having to taste what he was cooking did not help. He was putting on more weight than he realized. 'I did no exercise, and the bigger I got, the more I vegetated in front of the telly.'

When he moved house he registered with a new doctor who gave him a medical. The scales showed his weight at almost 19 stones (120kg). 'The nurse asked me to read the scales but I couldn't – my belly was in the way. There was no denying it – I was in bad shape. I was diagnosed with high blood pressure, high cholesterol, high everything. I knew I had to address my lifestyle now or I might not be able to see my daughters grow up.'

Gary was a binge-eater, eating six packets of crisps a day, numerous pies and pasties, pork scratchings, and a jumbo fry-up breakfast two or three times a week. He embarked on a three-year journey to lose weight. 'It was very hard in the early stages,' he admits, 'but then I saw the scales going down and that was the biggest motivator. My wife kept a chart of my progress, bought a vegetable steamer and lots of vegetables, and questioned every pasty I was tempted to eat.' His eating habits have changed dramatically. He now has a grapefruit and cereal for breakfast, a brown bread sandwich, cereal bar and fruit for lunch, and beans on toast for dinner. 'I still have a curry and a Sunday lunch once a week, because I believe it's important not to deprive yourself, but I was surprised to find I don't really miss the crisps and junk food.'

The doctor warned Gary not to exercise too hard initially, so he started taking regular walks, with a longer walk once or twice a week. His determination produced results: he lost 4 to 5lb (2kg) every week, until his weight levelled out after about 18 months. Gary joined a gym and started running. 'I am now down to 13 stone, my blood pressure and cholesterol are normal and I have challenged my brother to a half-marathon – and I think I have a good chance of beating him,' he says.

Adjusting your goals

Over the coming weeks and months, continue to keep track of the calories you consume and expend. Along the way, you may find you are losing weight steadily and then suddenly hit a plateau, when the pounds don't come off as easily or where your weight remains stuck where it is. Don't be discouraged. Almost everyone who has a significant amount of weight to lose hits a plateau.

The best advice, say experts, is to relax for a bit, celebrate the progress you've made and stick to your calorie goals. After a little while, the pounds may come off again. If not, increase the calories you burn by adding 15 minutes of exercise a day, or cut calories from your diet by eating less or eliminating a snack.

Once you reach your weight goal, you can adjust your diet again and gradually increase your calorie intake. This is because in order to lose weight, you must consume fewer calories than you need to force your body to burn fat for energy. To maintain your new weight, you need only to strike a balance between the calories you consume and those you burn. How much you increase your intake now depends on your ideal weight and how active you are. If you're a woman, try setting your maintenance level at 1,800 calories a day. If you're a man, set a goal of 2,100 calories a day. If you notice yourself beginning to gain weight, you'll need to increase your activity level or lower your calorie intake.

Don't be surprised if you need to adjust it again at some time. Most people who have successfully lost weight, especially those who have shed a great deal, say they have to continue to keep an eye on the calories they consume and push themselves to stay active. (That's why it's important that you really enjoy the form of exercise you choose – it's a long-term proposition!) And don't get too upset if you put on a few pounds when you are going through a bad time. You've lost the weight before, and you can do it again.

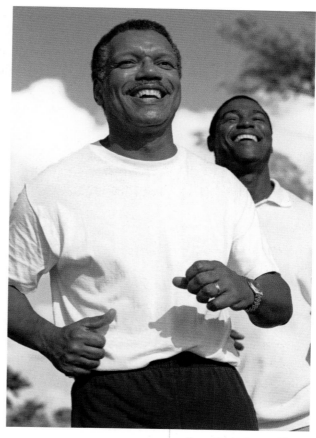

If you think of yourself as an active person who cares about eating well, you can use that new self-image to help you stay the course.

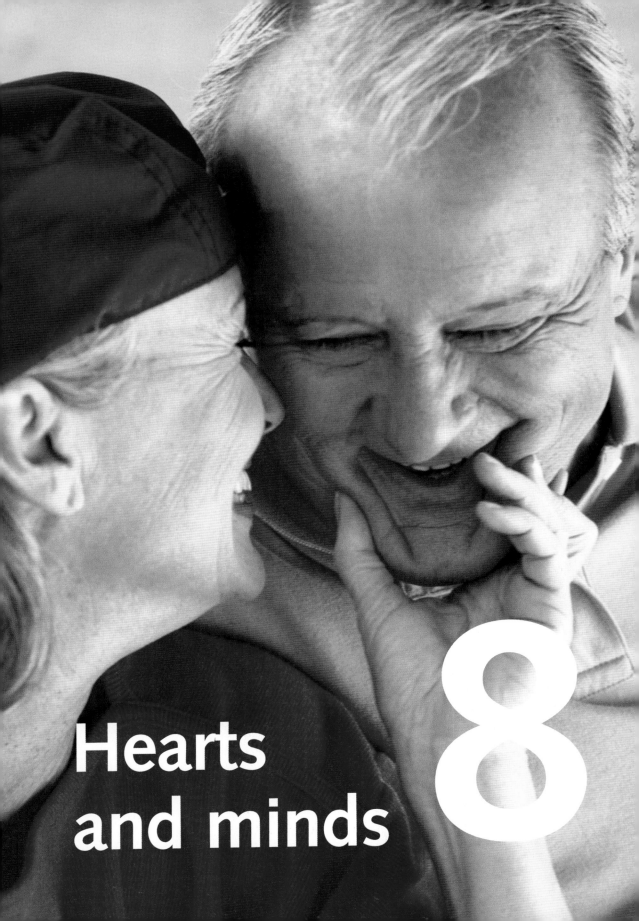

Hearts
and minds

8

The heart has long been linked with our emotions. When we're feeling sad, we say we're downhearted. When our feelings are there for everyone to see, we're wearing our heart on our sleeve. Now medical researchers have discovered powerful connections between our state of mind and the health of our heart. How does your outlook affect yours?

Dozens of studies have shown that negative emotions such as anger or depression increase heart disease danger. People suffering from depression may be as much as four times more likely than others to have a heart attack. Heart attacks also occur much more frequently in people coping with a divorce or separation. Anger and anxiety, too, seem to put a strain on the heart.

But if negative emotions threaten the heart, positive ones seem to protect it. People who are able to laugh at situations they encounter are at less risk of heart disease than those who rarely chuckle, according to findings published in 2001 in the *International Journal of Cardiology*. In another study, researchers looking at a group of almost 600 people with a family history of heart disease found that those who were optimistic were half as likely as their grumpier counterparts to develop heart problems.

Stress is hard on your heart

What forges the link between hearts and minds? Researchers don't have all the answers, but many believe that part of the connection is a physical reaction known as the stress response. When we're afraid or feeling threatened, our bodies go into high gear to prepare us for action. Our hearts begin to pound. Blood pressure increases. A hormone called adrenaline, which is a powerful stimulant, surges into the bloodstream. At the same time, glucose, fat and cholesterol are released into the blood in case we need extra energy. Chemical changes in the blood make it more likely to clot, possibly to reduce bleeding in the event of injury.

All these events are part of what psychologists call the fight-or-flight response. In the early days of human evolution, fighting or fleeing were usually the only choices we had in the face of danger. Even today, in situations of real physical danger, perhaps from a

> " **People** who are able to laugh at situations they encounter are at less risk of heart disease than those who rarely chuckle. "

Signs of stress

1 Fatigue
2 Frequent headaches
3 Insomnia or early wakening
4 Loss of appetite
5 Loss of sense of humour
6 Irritability or anger
7 Fidgeting or pacing
8 Increased eating or smoking
9 Blaming others
10 Shouting or swearing
11 Throwing things
12 Trembling hands

fire or a speeding car, the fight-or-flight response can be lifesaving. More often than not, the hazards we perceive are psychological, however. We worry about our jobs, our families, or our health – and these stresses can set off the same bodily reactions as those triggered by a physical threat. Researchers speculate that if we live in a constant state of worry or anxiety, the stress response can harm the heart. A racing heartbeat and elevated blood pressure may cause turbulence in the bloodstream that can damage artery walls, making them more vulnerable to the build-up of plaque, for example. The rush of glucose and cholesterol into the bloodstream may worsen the problem.

Both physical and emotional stress are known to trigger angina or even a heart attack in people with serious coronary artery disease because the combination of a pounding heartbeat and rising blood pressure increases the heart's need for oxygen. If coronary arteries are narrowed, they may not be able to supply the extra blood, and this can result in chest pain. Stress also triggers the release of fibrin, a substance that makes blood clot much more easily, and this could contribute to the formation of a clot in the coronary artery, causing a heart attack. Many people with coronary artery disease experience both angina and heart attacks during or immediately after periods of stress.

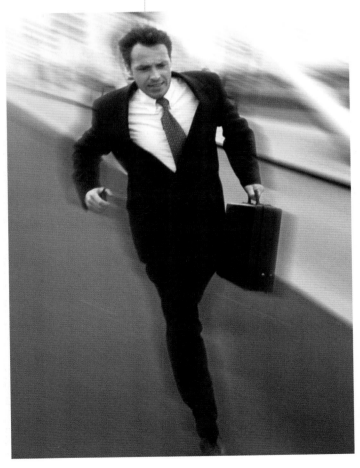

To test the link between anxiety and heart attacks, researchers at the University of California conducted a subtle experiment. They counted the number of deaths that occurred on the fourth day of each month, between 1973 and 1998. The fourth day was chosen because many Chinese and Japanese think that the number 4 is unlucky. (In Mandarin, Cantonese and

Are you a hothead?

Is the way you react to stress putting your heart at risk? Imagine yourself in the following situations. Even though they may not apply to your life, think about whether you might be likely to respond in the manner described.

● The appliance company promises to deliver your new dishwasher between 10am and noon, and now it's 2pm. You've called twice and left a message, and no one has called back. You can feel your heart racing and your stomach churning with anger.

Yes ■   No ■

● You've agreed to meet two friends for dinner before a concert, and they're already 15 minutes late. If they don't come soon, you may not have time to eat and get to the performance. You become so annoyed that when they finally arrive you can't relax enough to enjoy dinner.

Yes ■   No ■

● You're trying to get something done in your study, and your partner keeps coming into the room and interrupting you. Finally you've had enough, and you angrily demand to be left alone.

Yes ■   No ■

● Your boss criticizes you in front of colleagues. You're so angry that your hands are trembling and you can feel that you're perspiring. You even find yourself thinking of ways to get back at your boss.

Yes ■   No ■

● Just when you need a little support, your partner treats you coldly. Instead of saying something directly, you sulk silently about the way you've been treated and feel more and more resentful.

Yes ■   No ■

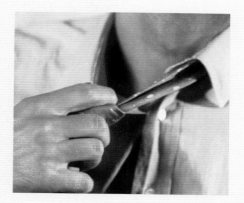

● Two friends you've invited to dinner call at the last minute to cancel, saying they're under the weather. The meal is almost prepared, the table is set. You can almost feel your blood pressure climb. You vow never to see these friends again.

Yes ■   No ■

● At the cinema, the couple in front of you keeps talking loud enough to disturb you. You could move to another seat. But their rudeness is so infuriating to you that you lean forward and angrily tell them to keep quiet.

Yes ■   No ■

● You're in the middle of a phone call when your friend puts you on hold to take another call. Thirty seconds pass, then a minute, and you can feel your irritation mounting. Finally you've had enough, and you slam the phone down.

Yes ■   No ■

Scoring: If you answered Yes to five or more of the statements, you may be what psychologists call a hot responder. Instead of remaining patient and calm, you react angrily, your heart rate accelerating and your muscles tensing. The more 'Yes' responses you circled, the more important it is for you to find ways to relax.

Japanese, the word for 'four' sounds almost exactly like the word for 'death'.) Sure enough, deaths from heart disease peaked on that day – but only among Chinese and Japanese people, not non-Asian Americans. For people of Chinese or Japanese ancestry who were in the hospital, the death rate was almost 50 per cent higher on the fourth of the month than other days. Even fears that most of us would think of as superstitious, it turns out, can increase the risk of a heart attack.

Is your personality putting you at risk?

All of us experience stress, of course, but not everyone develops heart disease as a result. Why do some people seem particularly vulnerable? Again, scientists don't have all the answers, but certain personality traits appear to increase the risk. The classic heart disease-prone personality is the Type A. Type A individuals aren't just ambitious, they're driven to succeed. And because they don't want anything to get in their way, they can be aggressive, even hostile. Type As are impatient, easily irritated and quick to anger. Always in a hurry, they often try to do more than one thing at a time. They talk on the phone while driving, for instance, or read reports while eating.

Some research suggests that Type As put a potentially deadly strain on their heart by pushing themselves and others so hard. In a study of 1,305 men, those who scored highest on a test used to measure Type A traits were three times more likely to have a heart

FAST FACT

The most commonly reported incident preceding a heart attack is an emotionally upsetting experience – particularly one involving anger.

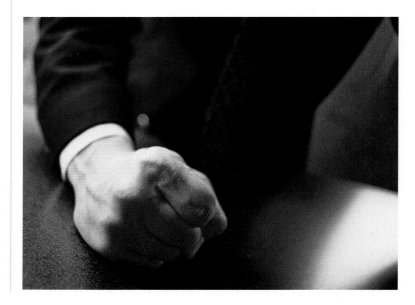

attack over the seven years that followed than men who scored at the bottom end of the scale. Although most studies of Type A behaviour have involved men, several investigations have looked at Type A women and found similar results.

By the 1980s, Type A behaviour was officially listed as an independent risk factor for heart disease, alongside elevated blood pressure and high levels of LDL cholesterol.

Hotheads, take note

However, many researchers aren't so sure, now, that Type A behaviour itself is the real problem. The true threat may be just one aspect of a Type A personality – hostility, or the tendency to react angrily, even at the slightest provocation. An anger-prone person is someone who gets right on the tail of a slow-moving car, hooting and even cursing. Or someone who lashes out angrily when a colleague arrives late for an important meeting because of an unavoidable delay.

▼ Key finding

The biological and psychological effects of stress were measured in a group of 183 men aged 45 to 63. The research team, based at University College, London, assessed changes to their nervous systems and measured their coronary heart disease risk factors, variations in their heart rate and cardiac activity. The men were also asked about their jobs, lifestyles, activity level and smoking and drinking habits. Results showed that the men who produced most stress hormones had abnormal heart rates and were more obese than the control group. Psychosocial factors such as job strain were thought to explain the increase in their production of the stress hormones that can affect the heart.

A 20-year observation of 1,400 men, looked at their obsessive habits, such as sticking to routines, disliking sudden change and being excessively meticulous. It also looked for signs of anxiety, such as sweating, sleep-disturbances and recurring indigestion. The London-based researchers found that the 127 men who died of heart attacks during the 20-year study had high scores for obsessive behaviour and anxiety symptoms.

A Welsh study of 2,890 men concluded that people who either openly expressed their anger or tried to suppress it were at an increased risk of heart attack.

Why is anger hard on your heart? One possible reason is that being constantly angry is stressful, increasing heart rate and blood pressure. But there may be other reasons. Ohio State University researchers recently found that men and women with high levels of hostility also had higher than normal levels of homocysteine, the

REAL PEOPLE, REAL WISDOM

Prayer for peace of mind

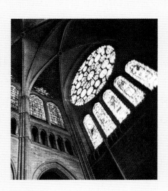

Yes, she knew her blood pressure was too high and her cholesterol levels were in the danger zone. But Josephine Richau was convinced the real reason she had heart disease was too much stress.

'I've always been a worrier,' says Josephine, an expert in special-education. In recent years she's had plenty of family problems to worry over. When things went wrong for one of her daughters a few years ago, Josephine and her husband found themselves raising one of their grandchildren — just when they'd planned to retire.

'Believe me, it hasn't been easy,' says Josephine. 'There are times when I've been under so much stress and pressure that I slip into a depression and have trouble getting out. Sometimes I can almost feel all the worry putting a strain on my heart.'

One day, rushing home to meet her husband, she started to feel a pain in her chest. It gradually subsided when she sat down and rested. But the next day, after experiencing another bout of crushing pain in her chest, she went to the hospital, where she was diagnosed with angina.

'The doctors gave me nitroglycerin pills to take. And for a little while I thought everything was back to normal,' says Josephine. 'But whenever I was under stress, I would experience more angina.' In the midst of giving a party for her grandson, she had another bout of chest pain, this time more severe than before. Back at the hospital, Josephine underwent an angiogram (an X-ray test that uses dye to create detailed images of the coronary arteries), which showed a severe blockage in one artery.

Today, thanks to an angioplasty, a procedure used to open up blocked arteries, she's feeling 100 per cent better. To stay that way, she tries to follow a healthy diet that includes more fruits and vegetables and to be as physically active as she can be. She's also making an effort to keep her weight down. 'But the most important thing I can do for my heart,' she says, 'is not become overwhelmed by stress, the way I used to.'

Josephine admits that's not easy. There are still days when the pressure of family problems leaves her feeling frazzled, and occasions when she gets depressed.

'But now, when things get bad, I try to slow down, take a deep breath, and put things in perspective. If it's something I can change, I try to change it. If not, I try to let it go.'

The most powerful antidote to stress, for Josephine, is prayer. 'Some people use a mantra. Some people meditate. I pray. I'm not overly religious, but I have a strong faith. I have a prayer that I say over and over when things get too pressured,' she says. 'It helps me to put all the worry aside and find strength when I'm feeling overwhelmed.'

blood chemical that is strongly associated with coronary artery disease. And in a University of Pittsburgh study published in 2001, researchers found that women who scored high on tests that measure anger had a fourfold or greater risk for high LDL and low HDL levels – both strong risk factors for heart disease. Anger has also been shown to make the blood more likely to clot.

The dangers of depression

People who are depressed or socially isolated are up to four times more likely to develop coronary artery disease. And once heart disease has set in, people who feel chronically depressed appear more likely to have a heart attack or die of their disease. Consider the results of a Swedish study that followed 275 men and women who had already had one heart attack. Those who scored high on tests that measure depression were three times more likely than more cheerful people to die of heart disease within a 10-year period.

No one knows exactly how sadness and despair wreak their havoc on the heart. Perhaps depression itself is stressful; or maybe depressed people are less likely to take care of themselves. A Dutch study looked at 2,900 people aged between 55 and 85, over a period of four and a half years. It found that in those who did not have heart disease, but who were depressed, death rates from heart disease almost quadrupled; and in those who already had heart disease, the death rate tripled. The British Heart Foundation observes that a patient who is severely depressed after a heart attack is three times more likely to have a second attack than one who is not depressed.

Symptoms of depression include persistent sadness, loss of interest in pleasurable activities, low energy, insomnia (especially early waking), weight loss or gain, difficulty concentrating, and loss of hope. If you think you might be depressed, talk to your doctor.

▼ Key finding

Sitting in a traffic jam for an hour may be enough to trigger a heart attack, say German scientists. In a study of 691 people who'd had a heart attack, 75 had been in traffic an hour or less before the attack and 175 had been exposed to traffic fumes in the previous three days. Taking diet and smoking habits into account, the researchers found that the risk of a heart attack tripled within the first hour of exposure to traffic fumes. Tiny particulates of soot from the fumes are probably to blame. Commenting on the findings, the British Heart Foundation agreed that increased pollution was probably the trigger – and drivers, cyclists and passengers on public transport are equally at risk.

Guarding your heart

Not every worrier or hothead is doomed to develop heart disease. And not everyone who lives a stressful life feels overwhelmed. But if your emotions are getting the better of you, it's time to act.

You can't change who you are, but you can change the way you react to events and situations. The first step is recognizing when stress is becoming a problem. And no one knows that better than you. If you're having trouble sleeping, if the simple pleasures of life don't give you much enjoyment anymore, and if you're tired much of the time, you may be suffering from chronic stress. (To rule out other health problems, mention your symptoms to your doctor.)

Next, identify the sources of the worst pressure and strain in your life. (If you feel anxious without really knowing why, and your feelings are so intense that they interfere with your daily life, you could be suffering from a condition known as generalized anxiety disorder, which can be treated with medication and/or with psychotherapy.) Then take some time to work out which ones you can eliminate or disarm.

> Sit down with your diary and find a way to rid yourself of the activities you can live without.

Facing stress head-on

If you're worried about money, take a hard look at ways to reorganize your finances or economize. If you and your partner are going through a rocky time, decide what steps you can take to alleviate the tension – then take them. You may find that making even one move toward alleviating the source of your stress can help to restore a sense of control over your situation and even galvanize you to make another one.

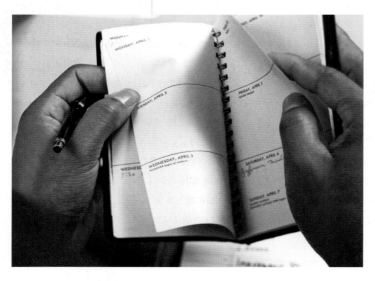

Being disorganized can cause a lot of aggravation if you can't find something when you need it. Regain control by setting up a filing system for your statements, accounts, paperwork, bills and letters, for instance. Deciding, once and for all, where to keep the car and house keys – and making sure they go there – can make everyday life a little less stressful.

If having just too many commitments is a problem, take charge of your time. Sit down with your diary and find a way to rid yourself of activities you can live without or delegate responsibilities that could be taken on by someone else.

Coping for the best

Of course, sometimes it's impossible to weed out the root causes of your stress. That's why it's also important to develop some coping skills. Remember, it's not a stressful situation that harms your health, it's your reaction to it. Here's how to get started.

1 Slow down The original term for Type A behaviour was 'hurry syndrome', because hard-driven people tend to do everything faster than more relaxed types. Encourage yourself to relax by consciously slowing your walking pace, driving more slowly and taking more time to enjoy your meals. The next time you find yourself rushing around, stop, take a deep breath and slow down.

2 Ease up on yourself Sometimes we put stress on ourselves by thinking in terms of absolutes, using words like 'never' or 'should' or 'always'. 'I should never have done that', we tell ourselves. 'She's always late whenever we need to be punctual.' If you notice yourself thinking in absolutes, lighten up. Replace

Smooth moves

Feeling stressed out? A yoga class could be the solution. Exercise scientists have long known that yoga offers a great way to stretch your muscles and improve your balance. Now psychologists are showing that it also eases a troubled mind. When researchers from the University of Würzburg in Germany tested 12 women before, during, and after a 60-minute yoga class, they found that the women's heart rates dropped dramatically during the class. The women also reported feeling less irritable. In fact, yoga may be one of the best ways to improve your sense of well-being. At Oxford University, a psychologist divided 71 men and women into three groups. One group practised simple relaxation techniques. The second used visualization to imagine themselves feeling less tense. The third did a half-hour yoga routine. The people in the first two groups reported feeling sluggish afterwards. The people in the yoga group, on the other hand, said they felt more energetic and emotionally content.

irrational thoughts with more reasonable ones. Things don't always go wrong for you, after all. The truth is, things occasionally go wrong for everyone. And when they do, everyone has the same challenge: to sort things out and get on with life.

3 Let it go Next time something gets you stressed or angry, take a step back and ask yourself if it's really worth getting worked up about. If it isn't, let it go. If you're a hothead, and you find your anger rising, count backwards from 10, then take a few deep breaths, concentrating on letting out a bit more of your anger each time you exhale.

The healing power of forgiveness

Most of us have been hurt by someone in our lives, and many of us have trouble letting go of that hurt. A cruel remark, a deliberately hurtful act, even physical violence, can all create lasting emotional distress. But new research suggests that nursing a grudge could put a strain on the heart. Releasing that anger by forgiving the person who hurt you could ease the burden.

The latest evidence comes from a study by researchers at Hope College in Michigan who asked volunteers to think about someone who had caused them pain. When the volunteers replayed in their minds the reasons they were angry and hurt, tests showed a sharp rise in their blood pressure, heart rate and muscle tension — the same psychological stress reactions that can trigger angina in people who have coronary artery disease and may even lead to artery damage in people who don't. But when those volunteers imagined themselves forgiving the person, tests showed a much less dramatic rise in signs of cardiovascular arousal.

No one has yet proved that people who tend to be more forgiving are less likely to develop heart disease, however — or that the act of forgiving someone will protect you from having a heart attack. But when researchers at the University of Michigan surveyed more than 1,400 people in 2001, they did find that people who said they'd forgiven someone who'd hurt them also reported being in better overall health than those who had never forgiven anyone.

'To err is human; to forgive, divine,' as the 18-century poet Alexander Pope wrote. That's still true today. In the University of Michigan study, only 52 per cent of respondents said they had forgiven someone who had hurt them. But 75 per cent believed that God had forgiven them for their own past wrongs.

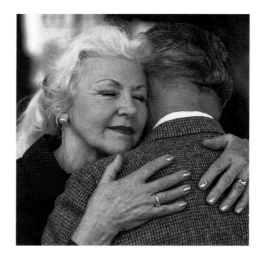

4 Distract yourself One of the simplest ways to banish nagging thoughts or sidestep anger is to put something positive in their place. Call a friend, put on a piece of music you love, take a hot bath or lose yourself in a good book. Engaging in a hobby that absorbs your full concentration is a perfect antidote to stress. For many, gardening can be especially therapeutic.

5 Get moving Several studies have found that physical activity helps to reduce stress and anxiety and may even be an effective

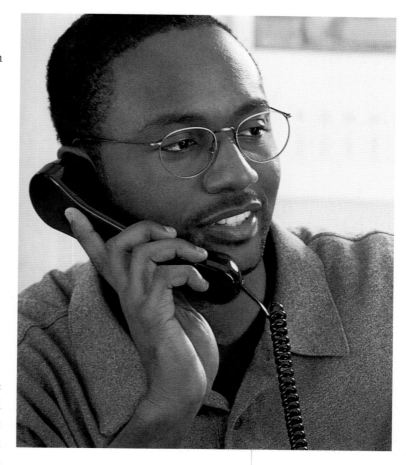

remedy for mild to moderate depression. In a 1998 study in which 38 men and 35 women kept diaries of activity, mood and stress, volunteers felt less stressed out on days when they were physically active than on those when they didn't exercise. Even when stressful events occurred, the participants felt less anxious on days when they were physically active. Exercise can also help to ensure that you get a good night's sleep, which can contribute to your well-being and make you feel better.

6 Call on a friend Spending time with someone you like does more than take your mind off your troubles – it could save your life. Swedish researchers recently reported that people with a strong sense of social connection to other people were almost one-third less likely to die in the aftermath of having a heart attack than those who were socially isolated. If you don't have a circle of friends to turn to, try building one by, say, volunteering for a local charity, becoming involved with your church or joining an environmental group that clears up riversides and open ground.

Worth a laugh
Looking for comic relief? Try one of these movies:

1 A Fish Called Wanda (1988)
2 Annie Hall (1977)
3 Bringing up Baby (1938)
4 Chicken Run (2000)
5 Dr Strangelove (1964)
6 Duck Soup (1933)
7 Monty Python and the Holy Grail (1975)
8 The Naked Gun (1988)
9 Shrek (2001)
10 Some Like it Hot (1959)
11 The Apartment (1960)
12 Airplane (1980)
13 The Producers (1967)
14 Tootsie (1982)
15 Toy Story (1995)

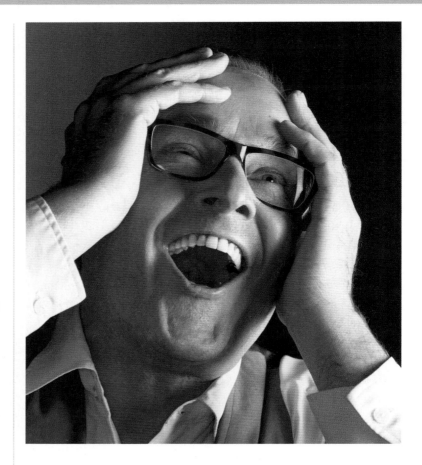

7 Have a good laugh Laughter, it's said, is the best medicine. In fact, being able to laugh at life's stresses could be an antidote to heart disease. In a study published in 2001, researchers tested 300 volunteers' propensity to laugh at everyday situations, surprise events or during encounters with friends. Those with a ready laugh were less likely to have coronary artery disease than those less apt to chuckle, the scientists found. Even among people with elevated blood pressure or cholesterol, the ability to laugh protected their hearts. If you can't seem to make light of the things going on in your own life, try renting an amusing video or reading a comic novel. A friend with a ready sense of humour, who can see the funny side of life will very often be able to help you to get back on an even keel.

The art of relaxation
You'd think relaxing would be easy. In fact, most of us have a hard time really emptying our minds and letting our bodies go limp. A little bit of practice can help. There are lots of ways to overcome worrying thoughts and soothe the spirit. Some people are drawn to

meditation or yoga. Others turn to prayer. The best method is simply one that allows you to find some quiet time away from the stresses of everyday life.

Relaxation is important not just to your emotional well-being but also to your health. Harvard University psychiatrist Herbert Benson was the first to measure the physical effects of relaxation techniques such as meditation. His discoveries surprised much of the medical community. By meditating, he found, people could actually lower their blood pressure, slow their breathing and reduce their body's oxygen consumption – controlling body functions previously thought to be entirely involuntary. In other words, while the body turns on the fight-or-flight response automatically, we can learn to turn it off, using the relaxation response. Eliciting the relaxation response is relatively simple. Just follow these steps.

1 Find a quiet place where you won't be disturbed. Sit in a comfortable position, one that will allow you to relax your body.

2 Close your eyes.

3 Breathe through your nose, concentrating on each breath. As you exhale, silently repeat a single word or short phrase, such as 'peace' or 'relax'. Choose something soothing.

4 Continue repeating your word or phrase and concentrating on your breathing for 15 to 20 minutes. (Don't set an alarm, or you'll constantly be thinking about when it will go off. Have a watch or clock handy and open your eyes now and then to check the time.)

5 Sit quietly for a few minutes, first with your eyes closed and then with them open. Enjoy the way your body and mind feel.

Whatever method you choose to activate the relaxation response, don't defeat the purpose by worrying whether you're doing it properly. The only measure of success is whether it helps you to relax. And don't give up if you find thoughts intruding. Just put them gently aside and refocus your attention on your word or phrase. The more you practise your relaxation technique, the more effective it will be.

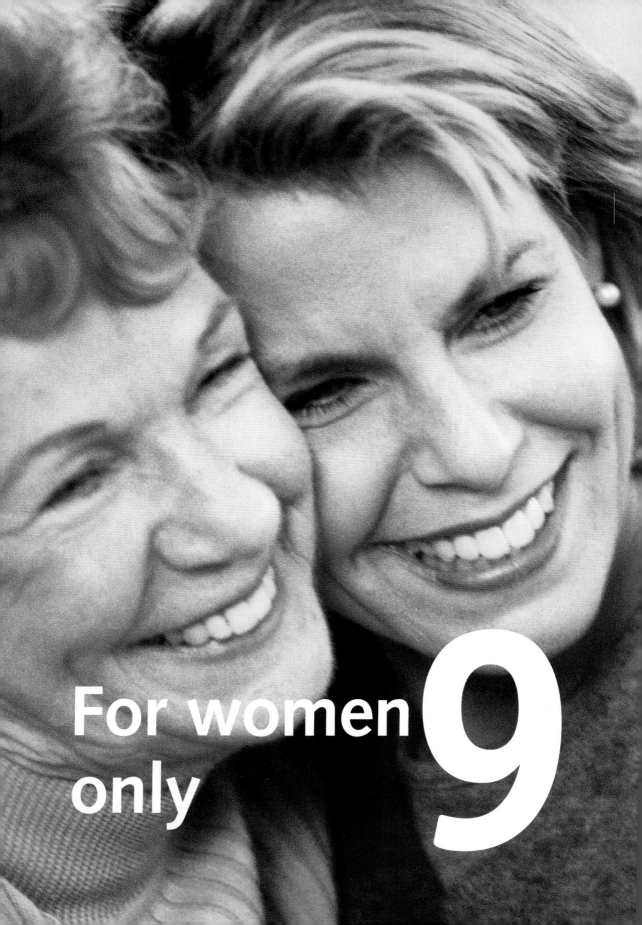

For women only 9

If you're like a lot of women, the most serious risk factor for heart disease you face is a false sense of security. Despite plenty of warnings to the contrary, many people still think of heart attacks primarily as a man's worry. That means they (and their doctors) are often slow to recognize the symptoms of trouble, with the result that women are dying of heart attacks that could have been prevented.

Heart disease is the leading cause of death for both sexes in the UK. It's true that men begin having heart attacks earlier in life than women do and until the age of 65 they suffer more of them. But once women have gone through the menopause, their risk of coronary artery disease begins to climb rapidly, catching up with that of men by the age of 65.

Crossing the gender gap

When researchers first began to look closely at the risk of heart disease in women, they turned up some surprising – and deeply troubling – facts. Among them:

- Women with symptoms of coronary artery disease typically wait longer than men do before they see a doctor.
- They tend to be sicker when they are finally diagnosed.
- They are treated less aggressively than men when they complain of heart disease symptoms. They are less likely than men to be given angiograms, for instance, tests that use injected dye to create an image of coronary arteries.
- Women under the age of 50 are more likely than men to die of a first heart attack.

The biggest discrepancy between the sexes is the age when heart disease first becomes apparent. Most women are protected until they go through the menopause. The reasons aren't entirely clear, although many experts believe that high levels of the female hormone oestrogen play a protective role. Oestrogen decreases LDL ('bad' cholesterol) and boosts HDL ('good' cholesterol). It also raises levels of a chemical called tissue plasminogen activator, or TPA, which dissolves clots. Moreover, prior to menopause, a

> "Once women have gone through menopause, their risk of coronary artery disease begins to climb rapidly."

woman's uterus churns out hormone-like chemicals called prostaglandins, which widen blood vessels and also help to prevent clots from forming. All these effects are likely to ward off heart disease and heart attacks.

As oestrogen levels dip after menopause, however, women's protection begins to vanish. By about 65 women have the same risk of coronary artery disease as men.

The fact that women develop heart disease later in life probably accounts for some of the differences in how the genders fare. Because women are, on average, ten years older than men when they are diagnosed, they tend to have more complicating conditions, such as diabetes, high cholesterol, or elevated blood pressure – conditions that make heart disease more dangerous. In 1999 Yale University researchers analysed data from 384,878 men

Test your knowledge on women and heart disease

What you don't know about heart disease can hurt you. That's especially true for women, who may delay seeing a doctor because they think they aren't at serious risk. Test your knowledge by ticking True or False, and then checking the answers.

● 1 The symptoms of a heart attack are always the same for women and men.
True ■ False ■

● 2 A heart attack is more than twice as likely to prove fatal for a woman under 50 than for a man of the same age.
True ■ False ■

● 3 Women are more likely to die of breast cancer than heart disease.
True ■ False ■

● 4 Among women, smoking causes just about as many deaths from heart disease as from lung cancer.
True ■ False ■

● 5 Hormone replacement therapy has been proven to lower women's risk of dying from a heart attack.
True ■ False ■

● 6 Hormone replacement therapy has been linked to an increased risk of breast cancer.
True ■ False ■

● 7 Diabetes poses a more serious risk to a woman's heart than to a man's.
True ■ False ■

● 8 Low levels of 'good' cholesterol pose a more serious risk to women than to men.
True ■ False ■

● 9 After 65 a woman's blood pressure is typically higher than a man's.
True ■ False ■

Answers:
1. False	4. True	7. True
2. True	5. False	8. True
3. False	6. True	9. True

and women who had suffered heart attacks. Almost 17 per cent of the women died while hospitalized compared with only 11.5 per cent of the men. But when the researchers accounted for the effects of age, the difference in death rates all but disappeared.

There was one exception, however. And it's a worrying one. Women under 50 who suffered a heart attack were twice as likely to die from it as were men of the same age. The younger that women were at the time of their first heart attack, the more likely it was to be fatal.

The reason is a mystery. The hazards of heart disease may be more serious in females than males simply because women's bodies – including their hearts and blood vessels – are smaller. Cholesterol build-up may be more dangerous in smaller arteries than in larger ones.

▼ Key finding

Many women don't take the threat of heart disease seriously, according to a 2003 report by the British Heart Foundation. Although cardiovascular diseases claimed the lives of 54,000 women in the UK in 2001 – more than four times the number dying from breast cancer – 40 per cent of the women questioned thought breast cancer the greater threat. Of those aged between 16 and 24, only 10 per cent said they feared cardiovascular disease, almost 50 per cent were concerned about lung and breast cancer. Perhaps most worryingly, 79 per cent of women have never discussed heart disease with a GP or practice nurse.

Similarly, coronary artery disease may be harder on a small heart than on a larger one.

But these differences don't explain all the seeming inequities between the sexes. The fact is, some doctors may be less likely to suspect heart disease in a female patient – especially those under 60. As a result, they may be less likely to order diagnostic tests such as stress tests or angiograms. One recent study found that angiograms were performed on 59 per cent of men with symptoms of coronary artery disease compared with only 53 per cent of women. A report from the British Heart Foundation found that although early studies show possible inequalities between men and women in assessment, diagnosis and treatment of coronary heart disease, these differences were very small, and reflected the women's increased age and medical history, which could have complicated both diagnosis and treatment.

The sad fact is that many younger women don't give their risk of heart disease a thought. At almost any age, women tend to be more preoccupied with breast cancer risk, even though the danger to their hearts is far more significant.

This is the bottom line: take the risk of heart disease seriously, and learn to recognize the symptoms of a heart attack. If you've already been diagnosed with coronary artery disease, take charge of your medical care by asking your doctor to discuss all the treatment options. If you're not comfortable with the advice and information you're given, ask to see another doctor.

Understanding a woman's risks

Although age difference is the most important distinction between the genders when it comes to heart disease, there are others. For instance, when men first develop symptoms of heart disease, they typically have one or two risk factors. Women are more likely to have multiple risk factors that together compound the danger. More women than men tend to be obese and have both high blood pressure and elevated cholesterol, for example. Being over-weight and having diabetes also seem to go hand in hand for many women.

Understanding the special concerns women face can help you to fine-tune your strategy for staying healthy. Here's what you need to know.

Diabetes In the UK, more women than ever are suffering from diabetes, increasing their risk of heart disease by at least three times. Diabetes UK reports that women with diabetes are eight times more likely to die of cardio-vascular diseases than women who do not have diabetes. This may be because they are more prone to the build-up of fatty deposits in their arteries. In addition, their blood clots more easily and they are more likely to have high blood pressure. All these factors put diabetics at much greater risk of cardiovascular problems than the average, non-diabetic woman.

Blood pressure High blood pressure increases heart disease risk in both men and women, but the problem may be more serious in women. In the UK, 40 per cent of women have high blood pressure and, by the time women reach 55, more than half have blood pressure high

FAST FACT

Contrary to the myth that it's a man's problem, cardiovascular disease (including heart attack and stroke) killed 12,000 more women than men in the UK in 2002.

Hot topic: Symptoms of their own?

Do men and women have different symptoms of heart attack? You would think so, reading some popular books and websites devoted to women's health. But focusing on the differences, some experts say, could be doing women more harm than good.

While it's true that a percentage of women, particularly younger women, experience atypical symptoms (instead of pain or pressure in their chests, they may feel only nausea or severe indigestion, along with shortness of breath, for instance), the number is quite small.

In the overwhelming majority, the symptoms are the same: pain or pressure in the middle of the chest, often radiating out down the left arm,

accompanied by sweating, nausea, or shortness of breath. By emphasizing gender differences in heart attack symptoms, critics say, some sources of health information may actually make women less alert to the most common indications of trouble.

For middle-aged and older women, the advice is simple: if you experience chest pain or pressure and/or shortness of breath especially during physical activity or emotional stress, call your doctor or dial 999 and chew an aspirin.

Don't wait. Studies show that women tend to put off seeing a doctor longer than men when the symptoms of coronary artery disease appear. That delay, for some, can prove fatal.

---

enough to put them in danger. After 65, women typically have higher blood pressure than men. The problem is more severe, in all ages, among Pakistani and Afro-Caribbean women.

Cholesterol Elevated LDL is dangerous for both sexes. But from 55 onwards, women's LDL levels tend to be higher than men's. Women may also be at greater risk when their levels of HDL cholesterol get low. In one recent study, low HDL was one of the most significant signals of increased heart disease risk in women, though not in men. (Elevated LDL appears to pose more danger in men than it does in women.) What's more, women seem to need slightly more HDL to ward off heart disease. The official guidelines for both sexes advise maintaining an HDL level of around 1mmol/l, but some studies show that women require a slightly higher level for protection.

Smoking Although smoking rates are declining among both sexes, the rate of decline is slower in women – more than 25 per cent of women in the UK still smoke. According to the British Heart Foundation, smoking carries almost twice the risk for the development of coronary heart disease in women as it does in men, and heavy smoking is the major risk factor for pre-menopausal CHD.

FAST FACT
There is an urgent need for women to address their risks. In 2003, a British Heart Foundation report on women in the UK found only 8 per cent named high cholesterol, 5 per cent named high blood pressure and 12 per cent named family history as factors which increase the likelihood of developing coronary heart disease.

Life-saving insights from America's nurses

In 1976 millions of women around the world were using oral contraceptives – potent drugs whose long-term effects had not been studied. To uncover any hidden health dangers, researchers at Harvard University contacted 170,000 nurses, asking them to fill out a questionnaire. Nurses were chosen in part because their medical expertise would make it easy for them to answer the brief but technical questions accurately. Some 122,000 people responded, and the Nurses' Health Study was born.

Recognizing that the nurses offered an unprecedented opportunity to study many aspects of women's health, the Harvard team began collecting more and more detailed information – about everything from smoking and hormone use to diet and exercise. Between 1982 and 1984 the study subjects even submitted 68,000 sets of toenail samples, which were used to analyse nutrient content in the diet. Even today, more than 25 years after the study started, 90 per cent of the questionnaires sent out every two years are filled in and returned.

Over that time, scientists have gained lifesaving insights into heart disease among women. The highlights include:

■ **The risks of being overweight** Nurses who gained 4 stones (25.5kg) over the course of the study period had more than five times the risk of developing high blood pressure. Overweight nurses who lost weight lowered their risk by 25 per cent.

■ **The benefits of physical activity** Walking at a pace of more than three miles an hour for at least one hour a week lowered the risk of stroke by about 30 per cent. Walking three or more hours a week, at a brisk pace, slashed heart disease risk by 35 per cent.

■ **The importance of whole grains** Women who ate at least one serving of whole grains a day cut their risk of ischaemic stroke by 30 to 40 per cent and their risk of diabetes by 25 per cent.

■ **The dangers of smoking** Heart disease is three times more prevalent among women who smoke than among nonsmokers.

■ **The risks of refined carbohydrates** Women whose diets were top-heavy with sugars and other highly refined carbohydrates had a two and a half times higher risk of heart disease than women who ate the lowest amounts of such foods.

■ **Snoring danger** Women who reported snoring were more than twice as likely to develop cardiovascular disease than those who didn't snore.

■ **The protective effects of fibre** Findings showed that eating one serving of a high-fibre breakfast cereal each day can cut heart disease risk by as much as 35 per cent.

Using a contraceptive pill Alarms sounded a few years ago when researchers linked oral contraceptives with a greatly increased risk of heart attack. According to several studies, women on the Pill were three to four times more likely to have a heart attack. But these numbers may not be as worrying as they seem. For a start, during childbearing years the overall risk of heart attack is very low, so the actual number of

▼ Key finding

Women are at greater risk of sudden and serious heart attacks during certain times of the month according to a small study of pre-menopausal women with heart disease symptoms. Among the 28 women studied, 20 reported developing heart-related problems within five days of beginning their menstrual periods, when oestrogen is at its lowest ebb.

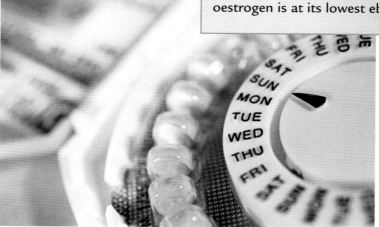

attacks linked to birth control pills is quite small. And newer oral contraceptives, which contain far less oestrogen than earlier ones, have been shown to pose virtually no risk. There is one exception. A 2001 study by researchers from Boston University School of Medicine found that the incidence of heart attacks was as much as 39 times higher than normal among heavy smokers on the Pill than among nonsmokers on the pill.

Being inactive and overweight More than seven out of ten women in the UK get barely any exercise at all; more than a third are overweight and 19 per cent are obese. Carrying excess weight raises heart disease risk for both men and women, but research suggests it increases more for women. Being sedentary more than doubles a woman's risk of dying from a heart attack.

Faulty diet and lack of exercise are the chief causes of obesity. So it's not hard to work out that making heart-healthy lifestyle changes may be even more important for women than it is for men.

4 THINGS TO KNOW ABOUT HRT

1 **HRT comes in many different forms**
Replacement oestrogen can be delivered via pills, patches, cream, and other methods. If you're considering HRT, talk to your doctor about the best choice for you.

2 **Many women experience side effects**
Although HRT eases some symptoms associated with menopause, it can also cause bloating, breast tenderness, cramping, spotting or a return to monthly bleeds.

3 **Dietary oestrogens may offer protection**
Some studies have shown that oestrogen-like substances, called phytoestrogens, found in soya and other plant foods may lower heart disease risk, although the evidence is controversial.

4 **New dangers may lurk**
The Million Women Study found that post-menopausal women on HRT were twice as likely to develop breast cancer as those not taking it.

Following a nutritious diet and getting moderate amounts of exercise on most days of the week are the most effective ways to keep many of these serious threats to your heart under control.

The HRT question

How safe is it to have HRT (hormone replacement therapy)? For millions of postmenopausal women, the issue of heart disease has come down to this one troubling question. At first, HRT promised to be a virtual fountain of youth, heading off not only heart disease but also many other age-related conditions.

Then came word that it can raise a woman's risk of breast cancer – and suddenly the potential benefits had to be weighed against a real risk. Now, new findings further complicate the issue. HRT can help to prevent osteoporosis in people who are unable to have other forms of osteoporosis-prevention, and is useful in cases of premature menopause (due to ovarian failure or surgery), it seems that power to prevent heart disease is not what researchers once hoped it might be.

From high hopes to nagging worries

It's easy to understand why cardiologists thought that taking oestrogen in the form of HRT might protect women's hearts. After all, as levels of the hormone fall in menopause, heart disease risk climbs. Taking synthetic oestrogen should, by all rights, extend the protection afforded by the natural hormone.

And indeed, early research findings augured well. Between 1987 and 1998 dozens of studies showed that women who took oestrogen after menopause had lower rates of coronary artery disease than those who didn't. In 1996, for instance, the Nurses' Health Study found that women receiving oestrogen were about half as likely as those not taking the hormone to develop the disease. Another study found that angina and heart attacks occurred 80 per cent less often in postmenopausal women on HRT.

Most of these studies were what researchers call observational studies. In other words, scientists simply observed large groups of women, including some who'd decided to take HRT. The trouble with such studies is that women who decide to take HRT may differ in other ways from those who don't. They may eat healthier diets, for instance, or get more exercise. The way around this is to do randomized studies, in which women are randomly assigned to receive oestrogen or a placebo and then followed to see how they fare. To almost everyone's surprise, the results of such studies for HRT have been disappointing. The Committee on the Safety of Medicines said in their 2003 update that in terms of heart disease, some HRT products that contain conjugated oestrogens do not prevent heart disease and may increase the risk of heart disease in the first year of taking them. The picture is still unclear with regard to other types of HRT.

The NHS's guidance to healthcare professionals is similar. They say that there is a possible risk of an increase in coronary heart disease in the first year of a combined HRT use. Oestrogen-only HRT does not seem to either increase or decrease the risk of coronary heart disease. They have come to the conclusion that there is no case for using HRT for primary or secondary prevention of coronary heart disease or stroke.

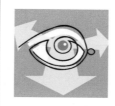

LOOKING AHEAD

SERMs – a safer alternative

An alternative to hormone replacement therapy is a non-steroidal compound that has an oestrogen-like effect on some tissues and an anti-oestrogenic effect on others. Called selective oestrogen receptor modulators, or SERMs, they are designed to stimulate only certain tissues, leaving others undisturbed. One SERM under investigation, called raloxifene, is already being used for the prevention and treatment of osteoporosis. Data on its effect on the heart is expected imminently, but it is already known to reduce overall cholesterol and LDL levels, while raising HDL levels.

Meanwhile, in a report from the Nurses' Health Study published in 2000, for example, scientists compared breast cancer risk in more than 46,000 women interviewed between 1973 and 1995. Women who were currently using HRT – or had used it sometime in the previous four years – were 20 to 40 per cent more likely to develop breast cancer than those not on therapy.

Then came the Million Women Study in which scientists at the Cancer Research UK Epidemiology Unit in Oxford analysed data from over a million women aged from 50 to 64, between 1996 and 2001. Half of them were using HRT or had done so in the past. The study registered 9,364 cases of invasive breast cancer and 637 breast cancer deaths. Researchers found that post-menopausal women using combination HRT were twice as likely to develop breast cancer as non-users, while the risk was 30 per cent among oestrogen-only HRT users. In all cases, the risk of breast cancer begins to decline when HRT is stopped. The latest UK advice is to use HRT for no more than five years.

What's a woman to do?

In the wake of the new data, many cardiologists have altered their advice to women. Hormone replacement therapy is no longer considered capable of protecting against heart disease. The results of ongoing studies may shed more light on the picture. But for now, here's what most experts say.

If you've been diagnosed with coronary artery disease, there's little evidence that starting HRT will help you to ward off a heart attack or slow the progress of the disease. And because studies show an increased risk of heart attacks during the first year on HRT, most experts now think the risks outweigh the benefits.

If you're healthy but want to reduce your risk of heart disease, don't rely on HRT. The Committee on Safety of Medicines says that HRT does not prevent heart disease and should not be used to protect against it. Meanwhile, there are more reliable ways to protect yourself, including exercise and a healthier diet.

What if you're currently on HRT? Should you stop? Talk to your doctor. If you've been on HRT for more than a year without any problem, you're probably past the period of increased heart attack risk. However, you should be on the lowest effective dose, and should come off it as soon as possible.

Of course, you still have to think about the issue of breast cancer. If the disease runs in your family, HRT may not be worth the added risk.

In reality, most women start using HRT to ease the symptoms of menopause, such as hot flushes, and many stop taking it within the first year because they don't like the side effects.

Tried-and-trusted tactics

Luckily, there are plenty of ways to prevent heart disease that are safer and more certain than hormone replacement therapy. Recent findings from the Nurses' Health Study show how powerful they can be.

During a 15-year period, scientists counted 1,128 heart attacks in a group of more than 84,000 women. Of those heart attacks, 82 per cent, the researchers concluded, could have been prevented if the women had followed basic heart disease prevention strategies. Those who most closely followed the familiar advice – to give up smoking, exercise at least 30 minutes a day and eat a high-fibre diet low in saturated fats and trans fats – were 80 per cent less likely than the others to develop heart disease.

> There are plenty of ways to prevent heart disease that are safer and more certain than hormone replacement therapy.

REAL PEOPLE, REAL WISDOM

Warnings you shouldn't ignore

'That's odd,' Sheila Schrier remembers thinking. Starting her regular workout on the treadmill at the fitness club, she felt unusually tired for the first five minutes. The feeling passed, though, and she didn't give it a second thought. She certainly never worried about her heart.

'My husband had had bypass surgery a few years before, and he'd had such a hard time of it,' says Sheila, 64. 'I was so preoccupied with his health that I never stopped to worry about my own. I knew that women get heart disease, but somehow I never really thought that could mean me.'

She experienced the same tiredness the next time she used the treadmill, so she thought she'd better see her doctor. And it's as well she did. An angiogram showed that a coronary artery was almost 90 per cent blocked.

'If I had a pound for every time someone said, "How could this happen to you?" I'd be a millionaire,' she says with a laugh. Slender and in tip-top shape, Sheila is the director of a fitness centre that specializes in cardiac rehabilitation programmes. Before her diagnosis she taught classes in water aerobics and also worked out several times a week. She had always eaten a healthy diet. Her cholesterol levels were normal. And although she had developed borderline high blood pressure after the menopause, she was taking a drug that brought it under control.

Her only real risk factor was a family history of heart disease: both her parents died of heart attacks. 'But they both smoked. They ate terrible diets. I was sure that by living a healthy life I'd be able to avoid that,' explains Sheila.

In fact, she did avoid a heart attack – by getting to the doctor in time, before the blockage cut off blood flow entirely. When an attempt to open up the blocked artery through angioplasty failed, Sheila underwent a coronary bypass, in which a new blood vessel, transplanted from another part of the body, is connected to supply the heart. Two months after the operation, she started a rehabilitation programme – as a patient this time. 'It wasn't easy,' she recalls. 'After the surgery, I was quite incapacitated. There were moments when I would suddenly feel panicky. It takes a while to get your energy back, and your confidence.'

A year later, she's back at work and even back to doing her own workouts, although not quite as strenuously as before. 'One thing I've come away from the experience realizing is how important it is to listen to your body,' she says. 'I think a lot of times when a woman complains about how she's feeling, there's a tendency for doctors to say, "Oh, it's all in her head." Fortunately, when something didn't feel quite right to me, I went to the doctor. I insisted that the tests be done. That may very well have saved my life.'

Taking your medicine

10

Researchers haven't yet devised a pill to cure heart disease, but they've won some very important victories. If you're at risk of heart disease but are still healthy, the latest medicines can help you to stay that way. If you've been diagnosed with coronary artery disease, new drugs can increase blood flow and ease the burden on your heart. Even during a heart attack, that old medicine-chest standby, aspirin, has been proven to help to limit the damage to the heart. Meanwhile, sophisticated 'super aspirins' that offer even more powerful heart protection have come along.

One of the biggest challenges cardiologists face is getting people to take their medicines. Failure to use drugs as directed is a growing problem. The more effective a heart disease medication is, the more important it is to take it as prescribed. Fail to take it, and you could be depriving yourself of lifesaving benefits.

Taking the risk out of risk factors

One of the most important advances in recent years has been the development of new drugs for conditions that increase heart disease risk, such as elevated cholesterol and high blood pressure. UK heart experts say that an estimated 15,000 heart disease deaths could be prevented each year in the UK, if everyone with cholesterol levels in the danger zone were taking them. In the USA, the latest generation of cholesterol-lowering drugs has been shown to slash the risk of heart attacks by 30 per cent in people with raised cholesterol. Even people with only moderately elevated cholesterol levels could benefit from these medications, recent evidence suggests. If that's true, many Britons might do well to begin drug therapy. Yet barely 35 per cent of those who could most benefit from these drugs are actually taking them.

One reason for this is lack of knowledge. There are still plenty of people around who don't know that their cholesterol levels are too high. Critics blame doctors for not being pro-active enough in

> " In the USA, the latest generation of cholesterol-lowering drugs has been shown to slash the risk of heart attacks by 30 per cent in people with raised cholesterol . "

testing their patients or prescribing the medications. Even when doctors prescribe the drugs, though, many people don't follow their orders. Studies show that as many as half the patients prescribed statin drugs, such as Lipitor (atorvastatin), stop taking them within the first year. The same problems limit the effectiveness of other potentially lifesaving drugs, including those that control blood pressure and diabetes.

The cholesterol tamers

Moderately elevated cholesterol can often be brought under control with a healthier diet that's low in saturated fat and abundant in high-fibre foods. But not everyone's cholesterol responds to dietary changes. Some people have cholesterol so high that even the best diet can't bring it back down to earth. Fortunately, a variety of medications can do the trick safely and effectively. They are:

Statins (HMG-CoA reductase inhibitors) The newest cholesterol-fighting medications, statins lower cholesterol levels by blocking an enzyme in the body that is needed to make cholesterol. Statins reduce both LDL cholesterol and triglyceride levels and raise HDL levels slightly.

In 2003, a UK trial of nearly 6,000 people in 69 hospitals provided definitive evidence that statins cut the risk of heart attacks and strokes by about a third in diabetic patients, irrespective of any existing arterial disease. Lowering cholesterol with 40mg of simvastatin was effective in all types of diabetic patient, and was not affected by the patients' age, sex or cholesterol level.

FAST FACT

More than 1.8 million people in the UK are now receiving statins, and it is thought that this saves 6,000 to 7,000 lives a year.

Are statins safe?

If you're taking a cholesterol-lowering statin, you may have heard that one such drug, sold under the name Lipobay (cerivastatin), was taken off the market. In August 2001 it was announced in the USA that the drug's manufacturer was voluntarily withdrawing the medication after 31 Americans taking it died due to rhabdomyolysis, a severe problem that results in the breakdown of muscle cells.

Other statins have also been associated with rhabdomyolysis, but the problem is very rare among users of these forms of the drug. Lipobay (Baycol in the USA) was withdrawn only when reports suggested a higher risk to users. Experts say the very real benefits of cholesterol-lowering statins – including a dramatically reduced threat of heart attacks – far outweigh the very small dangers.

Now that experts have revised the recommended levels of LDL and HDL cholesterol, you may be a candidate for statin drugs even if you weren't before. According to the British Heart Foundation, you're a candidate for drug therapy if:

- You're at very low risk of coronary artery disease, but your LDL cholesterol is 4.8mmol/l or higher
- You have two or more risk factors for coronary artery disease, and your LDL cholesterol measures 4.1mmol/l or higher
- You have coronary artery disease, and your LDL cholesterol measures 3.3mmol/l or higher

▼ Key finding

If you are taking a statin drug, you may want to think twice before taking antioxidant supplements such as vitamins C and E. In a study published in November 2001 in *The New England Journal of Medicine*, researchers found that antioxidants blunted the effectiveness of the statin drug Zocor (simvastatin) in people who were also taking niacin. The scientists measured the rate of atherosclerosis in 160 patients. Blockages decreased slightly in those taking the two drugs; but they increased by 0.7 per cent in patients who took antioxidants as well.

Because statins are processed in the liver, doctors usually recommend periodic blood tests to check how your liver is functioning. Examples of statin drugs available in the UK include Lipitor (atorvastatin), Zocor (simvastatin), Lescol (fluvastatin), Crestor (rosuvastatin) and Lipostat (pravastatin).

Bile acid sequestrants Like statin drugs, bile acid sequestrants help the body to get rid of LDL cholesterol. Studies show that these drugs lower LDL levels by about 10 to 20 per cent. Bile acid sequestrants usually come in a powder that has to be mixed with water or juice. Examples include Questran (cholestyramine) and Colestid (colestipol hydrochloride).

Niacin (nicotinic acid) Niacin, a form of B vitamin, was one of the first cholesterol drugs, and doctors still prescribe it, specially for patients with low levels of 'good' cholesterol. This is because it is one of the only drugs that significantly boosts HDL. On average, niacin reduces LDL cholesterol by 10 to 20 per cent, decreases triglycerides by 20 to 50 per cent and boosts HDL by 15 to 35 per cent. The only reason that niacin is not prescribed more often is that it can cause uncomfortable side effects, including nausea, indigestion, wind, vomiting and diarrhoea, as well as liver problems, when people take too much too quickly. Patients are usually started on a low dose which is gradually increased to more effective levels, to give the body time to get used to it.

Blood pressure medications

Even a small reduction in blood pressure can make a big difference to your health. One recent study showed that bringing diastolic blood pressure (the bottom number) down just 6mm/Hg reduced death from heart attacks by 14 per cent and strokes by 42 per cent. For some people, exercise and a low-salt, high-fibre diet will do the trick, but if not, there are drugs that can safely rein in elevated blood pressure. The most common categories include:

Diuretics Sometimes called water pills, diuretics work in the kidneys, flushing extra water and sodium out of the body and so reducing the amount of fluid in the blood. One of the most commonly prescribed is bendroflumethiazide.

Calcium–channel blockers These drugs relax the arteries to lower blood pressure and are considered very effective, especially for people with very high blood pressure. (See also page 182.)

Beta-blockers Beta-blockers bring down blood pressure by blocking nerve impulses to the heart and blood vessels, making the heart beat more slowly and with less force. Beta-blockers are sometimes used to restore normal heartbeat rhythm to people with some types of arrhythmia. Examples used in the UK include Inderal (propranolol), Betaloc (metoprolol) and Tenormin (atenolol).

Alpha-blockers Alpha-blockers reduce another form of nerve impulse to blood vessels, allowing blood to flow through more easily and so reducing blood pressure. Examples include Cardura (doxazosin), Hypovase (prazosin) and Hytrin (terazosin).

Alpha-beta-blockers This combined drug relaxes blood vessels and slows heartbeat. The result: Less blood is pumped through vessels, and blood pressure falls. One commonly prescribed alpha-beta-blocker is Trandate (labetalol).

ACE inhibitors Angiotensin-converting enzyme inhibitors block the production of the hormone angiotensin II that causes blood vessels to narrow. With less of the hormone in the body, they remain open, and blood pressure falls. Examples include Capoten (captopril), Innovace (enalapril) and Zestril (lisinopril).

Angiotensin receptor blockers A new alternative to ACE inhibitors, ARBs directly block the hormone angiotensin II from binding to blood vessels and thereby constricting them. Some

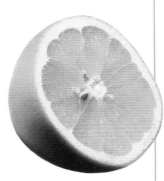

patients experience fewer side effects with angiotensin receptor blockers than with ACE inhibitors. Examples include Aprovel (irbesartan), Cozaar (losartan) and Amias (candesartan).

Vasodilators These drugs work directly on the muscles in blood vessel walls, relaxing them. As blood flows more easily, pressure drops. Examples of vasodilators available in the UK are Apresoline (hydralazine) and Loniten (minoxidil).

Don't be surprised if your doctor prescribes two or more blood pressure medications. Most patients who need drug treatment for raised blood pressure actually require a combination of two or more drugs for the best control, largely because many of these drugs work best in combination. And you may find that your doctor has to tinker with the combination to get it just right – or change it over time as your blood pressure changes. It sometimes takes a little while for doctors to hit on just the right prescription. If you experience symptoms like dizziness or coughing (a possible side effect of ACE inhibitors), be sure to mention them to your doctor.

Easing the burden on ailing hearts

If you've already been diagnosed with coronary artery disease, several drugs can help to ease the strain on your heart and relieve angina, the chest pain or pressure that occurs when blocked coronary arteries make it hard for the heart to get the oxygenated blood it needs.

Angina medications work by increasing blood flow through obstructed arteries or by reducing the heart muscle's need for oxygen, or both. If your angina is mild or you have the symptoms only now and then, your doctor may recommend a drug to take when you feel the problem coming on. If you experience angina regularly, your doctor may recommend a drug that you take every day. Medications to treat angina include:

Nitrates (nitroglycerin) Nitrates have been used for more than a century to relieve angina, and they are still among the most common drugs prescribed.

They work by widening blood vessels, making it easier for oxygenated blood to reach the heart. Nitrates come in tablet, spray or patch form. Usually the tablets are dissolved under your tongue or between lip

TROUBLESHOOTING TIP

If you have angina, keep a nitroglycerin spray on hand in case you experience chest pain. It is more stable than nitroglycerin tablets which lose their effectiveness six weeks after the bottle has been opened. The drug is also sensitive to light and moisture, so don't leave the container in a sunny place and don't store it in the bathroom or refrigerator.

and gum so the active ingredients reach the bloodstream rapidly. If you are using the spray, it is most commonly administered under the tongue.

Nitrates can be used when you are having an angina episode or if you are about to encounter a situation that typically triggers one, such as physical activity or a stressful event. The drugs work very quickly, usually within three to five minutes. In some cases you may need to take more than one pill. If the pain hasn't gone away after 15 minutes, call an ambulance to drive you to the nearest accident and emergency department.

Calcium-channel blockers Calcium-channel blockers interrupt the ability of calcium molecules to enter muscle cells in the heart and blood vessels. The result is that the heart rate slows, and the

Hot topic: Taking a pill vs making a change

With all the talk of cholesterol-lowering drugs, it's easy to wonder what ever happened to making changes to your lifestyle, like getting more exercise and eating a healthier diet. Weren't they supposed to rein in runaway cholesterol and keep blood pressure from going too high?

Indeed, some experts worry that we may rely too much on medicines and not enough on leading healthier lives. Reports suggest that some people taking medications, such as statins, actually begin to ignore advice about healthy eating, convinced that the drugs will make up for the shortcomings of their diets.

The truth is, keeping to a healthy diet and getting plenty of exercise are still the most reliable ways to reduce your chances of having a heart attack. Drugs that improve cholesterol levels or tame high blood pressure are only a second line of defence, when lifestyle changes don't work. But there's plenty of evidence that they usually do. One study found that volunteers dropped their LDL levels by an impressive 33 per cent by following a diet low in saturated fat and high in fruit and vegetables. A combination of exercise and a high-fibre, low-fat diet has been shown to bring moderately elevated blood pressure back down into the safe zone – without the help of any drugs.

Not surprisingly, however, people in the real world aren't usually as successful at making lifestyle changes as volunteers taking part in well controlled studies. No one likes to admit it, but it is easier for many people to pop a pill than to change their eating and exercise habits.

It's important to remember that pills never replace the need to make lifestyle changes. Even if you do have to take drugs for cholesterol or blood pressure, it's still important to give your medicine some help. The more you improve your health through diet and exercise, the less medication you'll need, and the healthier your heart will be, since diet and exercise provide a host of other benefits that no pill can offer.

strength of the contractions diminishes, reducing the heart's oxygen needs. Calcium channel blockers also widen blood vessels and lower blood pressure, making it easier for the heart to pump blood through the body. Examples include Tildiem (diltiazem), Istin (amlodipine) and Adalat (nifedipine).

Beta-blockers The same drugs that are used to lower blood pressure can also help to treat angina. Beta-blockers slow the heartbeat and reduce blood pressure, particularly during physical activity, making it possible for people with angina to exert themselves more before developing chest pain. These drugs have been shown to cut the risk of having a second heart attack in half and to lower cardiac mortality rates by 20 per cent.

An aspirin a day?

After years of being used to ease aches and pains, aspirin has recently been found to offer powerful protection against heart attacks. Aspirin works by thinning the blood so that clots can't form as easily.

The best evidence for the heart benefits of aspirin is in people already diagnosed with coronary artery disease. If you've had a heart attack, taking aspirin will help to prevent the formation of new blood clots that might lead to a second attack. If you've had coronary bypass surgery, taking aspirin will lower the chances that your new arteries will become blocked with clots. If you're having a heart attack, putting an aspirin under your tongue sends anti-clotting substances into the bloodstream that can dissolve the clot and dramatically reduce the risk of heart muscle damage.

The humble aspirin has been known, for at least a decade, to prevent heart attacks and strokes in thousands of people with a high risk of cardio-vascular disease, but it is massively under-used, according to research published in the *British Medical Journal*. Studies show that aspirin could prevent at least 7,000 deaths a year, but that fewer than half the patients with high-risk conditions are prescribed aspirin, and an extra 3,000 lives a year could be saved, in the UK, if everyone with a high-risk condition (for whom aspirin was appropriate) received it.

But what if you don't have heart problems? Can aspirin lower your risk of developing coronary artery disease? The British Heart Foundation says the evidence isn't clear. Most experts do not recommend that people free of heart disease take aspirin to lower their risk – partly because the evidence of benefits is uncertain and partly because taking aspirin daily or even every other day can irritate the stomach lining and cause gastrointestinal bleeding. And it can cause problems if you're already taking a blood-thinning medication or if you have asthma.

If you have heart disease, ask your doctor about taking aspirin. The latest evidence suggests that a very small dose, just 75mg – roughly a quarter of one standard adult tablet – is enough to protect your heart. So, most specialists recommend taking a baby aspirin, which contains roughly the same dose.

TROUBLESHOOTING TIP

If you're taking aspirin to prevent a heart attack, what should you take for pain? Not ibuprofen (the pain reliever found in Advil and Nurofen). The Medicines Monitoring Unit at Dundee University found a potentially serious interaction between low-dose aspirin and ibuprofen. The study found that cardiovascular patients taking both were twice as likely to die as those taking only aspirin. Preparations containing paracetamol (such as Panadol) are a better choice.

Beyond aspirin

New drugs are available that are even more powerful than aspirin: they can break up life-threatening blood clots and help to prevent new ones from forming. Every year, thousands of people survive heart attacks that might have been fatal, thanks to such medications. The drugs are also prescribed after procedures such as angioplasty and bypass surgery to ward off new blockages. Here are the main types:

Thrombolytics Usually administered intravenously during a heart attack, these drugs dissolve clots in arteries that supply both the lungs and the heart. In about 80 per cent of heart attack patients who are given a thrombolytic drug within 2 hours of warning symptoms, blood flow is restored. Examples include Streptase (streptokinase), Actilyse (alteplase) and Metalyse (tenecteplase).

Anticoagulants As the name suggests, anticoagulants help to prevent blood from coagulating or clotting, by reducing the amount of protein in the blood that is involved in clotting. Some anti-coagulants are administered by injection, others in pill form. They are usually prescribed after a heart attack or an angioplasty to reduce the chances of new clots forming. They are sometimes also used to prevent clots in people with heart failure. (If the pumping action is weak, the blood flow is sluggish, increasing the likelihood of clots.) Drug examples include warfarin, Clexane (enoxaparin) and Calciparine (heparin).

If you're taking a blood thinner, talk to your doctor before taking aspirin, vitamin E or fish oil, which also thin the blood. The combination of these with a blood thinner could be dangerous.

Super aspirins These drugs work like aspirins do – by inhibiting the function of platelets, which are blood cells involved in clotting. One such drug is Aggrastat (tirofiban). It's modelled on a venom used by the African saw-scaled viper. The venom contains a protein that prevents platelets in the blood from clumping together, causing the victim to bleed to death. Aggrastat is often prescribed for patients with unstable angina.

Another super aspirin, called Plavix (clopidogrel) has been in wide use in the UK for some time. Like anti-coagulants, super aspirins are usually prescribed to patients who have had a heart attack or undergone an angioplasty or angiogram.

Drugs only work if you take them

Although researchers have been able to create dozens of lifesaving heart medications, they haven't found a way to do something much more basic but equally important: to get patients to take their medicine as directed.

Studies show that fewer than half of all prescriptions are taken according to the directions on the label. Some patients skip a dose now and then, or they take it at the wrong time. Others go off a medication when they think they don't need it anymore. In one

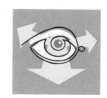

LOOKING AHEAD

Gene therapy for heart attack protection

Intensive research is under way to understand the genetic basis of heart disease – research that could yield new treatments in the form of gene therapy.

In a preliminary study, scientists at the University of Arkansas recently tested a genetic approach to limiting heart muscle damage during heart attacks. When blood supply to the heart is cut off, blood levels of a protein called angiotensin-converting enzyme, or ACE, rise steeply. This worsens heart muscle damage. To counter the destructive effect, researchers designed a strand of DNA that attaches to the gene that controls the production of ACE protein, blocking it. In animal studies this approach was shown to protect the hearts of rats during heart attacks. Trials in humans are the next step.

recent study, 85 per cent of patients who had been prescribed a heart drug were no longer taking it after two years. Other research shows that some people never even fill their prescription.

The problem of noncompliance – failing to follow doctors' orders – costs thousands of lives a year. Statins alone could save up to 15,000 lives annually in the UK. Yet in a study of individuals given prescriptions for one of these drugs, only one in five patients was still taking the pills as directed after a year.

Noncompliance is one reason a shocking 82 per cent of people with coronary artery disease – those at high risk of a heart attack – still have cholesterol levels in the danger zone. Even many heart attack survivors fail to take clot-dissolving medications as directed, drastically increasing their risk of a second heart attack.

The news is no better in terms of high blood pressure, either. More than sixteen million people in the UK suffer from high blood pressure, yet most people don't know they have it. According to the British Heart Foundation, three-quarters of those who have high blood pressure are not being treated; and of those who are treated, only 40 per cent have their hypertension under control.

Excuses, excuses

Why do so many of us ignore our doctors' orders? Researchers who study the problem of noncompliance have heard every excuse in the book from patients they've interviewed. Here are some common ones – along with good reasons not to skip those pills.

'I didn't think I needed the medication any longer.' When a drug makes you better, many people feel that they don't need it any longer. They are dangerously wrong about this, because drugs to control blood pressure or cholesterol typically have to be taken for years, even for the rest of your life.

In a recent Scandinavian study, 30 per cent of patients who stopped taking their cholesterol-lowering drugs said they did so because their cholesterol levels were now 'normal'. What they don't realise is that when the drugs are stopped, cholesterol levels often climb back up.

▼ Key finding

If you want to live longer, make sure you take your cholesterol-lowering medicine. According to findings from the West of Scotland Coronary Prevention Study, patients who took 75 per cent or more of the recommended doses of a cholesterol-lowering drug cut their risk of premature death by one-third more than those patients who took less than 75 per cent of the pills they had been prescribed.

'I was never really convinced the medicine worked in the first place.' To take a drug regularly, every day or even several times a day, you've got to be convinced that it's doing you some good. If you're not sure you really need the medicine your doctor has prescribed, say so right away. Ask your doctor what the medicine is supposed to do and what evidence there is that it works. The more you know about the benefits and side effects of a drug, the more likely you are to stick to the regimen.

'I'm worried about the side effects.' Many of the newest heart disease drugs have fewer and less serious side effects than earlier ones. Still, potent drugs often have some side effects. Talk to your doctor about what to expect. If you notice symptoms that worry you after you start on a drug, call your doctor immediately. In some cases, side effects go away as your body gets used to the medication. If they don't, your doctor may be able to switch you to a different drug or prescribe something that will counteract the side effects.

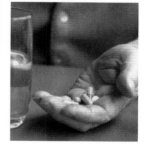

'I have trouble remembering to take a drug more than once a day.' This is a very common problem. Studies show that compliance falls off steeply when patients are asked to take a drug more than once a day – and it's not surprising. It's simple enough to remember to swallow your pills every morning. But if you have to take one at noon and another in the evening, it's easy to get distracted and forget. If that is happening to you, ask your doctor if another drug is available that can be taken only once a day. Otherwise, turn the page for some ways to help you to stick to your regimen.

'I never thought the problem was that serious in the first place.' This is another one of the top reasons people don't follow their doctors' advice. Of course it's easy to think elevated cholesterol or high blood pressure isn't that serious, since neither usually has symptoms. If you're not convinced the problem is worth treating, ask your doctor to explain why he or she thinks it's important to take a medication. Better still, do some reading of your own. Your local library or the internet will have plenty of useful information. Try to base your decisions on facts, rather than hiding behind ignorance.

TROUBLESHOOTING TIP

Whenever you pick up a prescription from a pharmacy, double-check to make sure you're getting the right drug in the right dosage. When researchers analysed 9,846 prescriptions filled at a large hospital's outpatient pharmacy in New Jersey, they found 1,371 mistakes, ranging from bottles containing the wrong pills or the wrong dosage to labelling errors. When in doubt, ask the pharmacist to double-check your prescription. And if the name doesn't match what was on the prescription form, ask why.

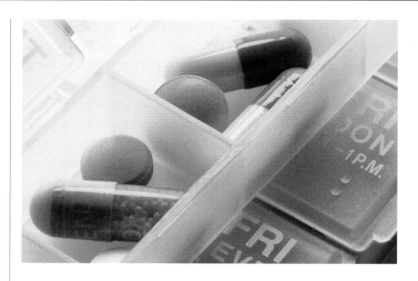

Tips for minding your medicine

Not everyone deliberately skips pills or neglects to refill their prescriptions, of course. More often, people just forget. Especially if you have to take a prescribed drug several times during the day – or several medications that have different schedules – it's easy to become confused and miss a dose or two. Studies have shown that the more drugs people are taking, the more likely they are to run into trouble following directions. If that sounds like you or someone you know, these simple tips can help.

- Take all your one-a-day medicines at the same time every day so you'll be less likely to forget.
- Time your pill-taking with something else that's part of your everyday routine – brushing your teeth, for instance, or eating breakfast (as long as you can take your pills with food).
- Use a pill organizer, available at most pharmacies or through mail-order catalogues. Choose one that you can open and close easily and that contains enough compartments for the various pills you take. Some let you set out a week's worth of pills and even provide different compartments for pills taken at different times of day.
- If you have a personal computer, programme it to give you a daily reminder. Most calendar and scheduling programs will buzz or beep or post an on-screen reminder. These are particularly useful if you work on your computer or check your e-mail several times a day. Of course, you can always set an old-fashioned clock radio or alarm to remind you when it's

time to take your pills. Reset it after it rings if you have to take pills more than once a day. It may irritate you so much that, in sheer self-defence, you start remembering to take them, unaided.

- Call your own answering machine and leave a message reminding you to take your medicine. Don't erase it. That way, every time you check your messages, you'll be reminded.
- Leave yourself a message on the refrigerator door, or beside your favourite armchair.

Hi-tech reminders

Some people need more than just a note on the fridge to help them remember to take their medicine. If you're one of them, there are several types of product on the market that can help. Some of these clever devices can be found in chemists. Or order one on-line at a website such as www.medicalarm.co.uk For more information, talk to your doctor or pharmacist.

■ Automated pillboxes
Instead of a container that merely holds your pills, how about one that reminds you to take them? Automated pillboxes are available that vibrate, sound an alarm or offer spoken reminders when your medicines are due. More expensive models automatically dispense pills, opening the appropriate compartment when it's time to take them. Cost depends on size and how fancy the system is.

Basic models cost as little as £10; the fanciest as much as £100.

■ Pocket dispensers These handy little containers, which fit in your pocket, carry a day's worth of tablets and beep when it's time to take them.

■ Mobile phone reminder You can set your mobile phone to beep or ring at certain times of the day, to remind you to take your medication.

■ Watches Specially designed watches not only tell the time but also beep, flash or vibrate when it's time for your medicine. Some even display the name of the pill to take.

■ Messaging services Still in the pipeline (but already available in the USA) is a messaging facility that calls you to remind you to take your pill. Some can even alert your chemist that your supply of pills is running low.

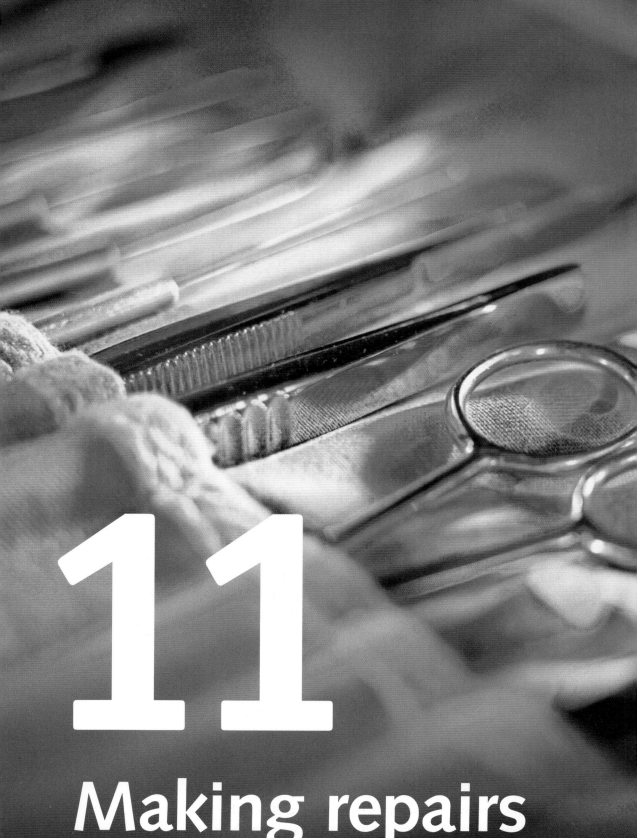

11
Making repairs

In 2001, a thrilling medical achievement took place: the implanting of the first self-contained mechanical heart inside the chest of a desperately ill man. With less publicity, many other advances in the field of cardiac surgery have made it possible for surgeons to mend damaged hearts and unclog blocked arteries – bringing new hope to hundreds of thousands of heart patients every year.

It's now routine for surgeons to take blood vessels from one part of the body and reconnect them near the heart to bypass blocked coronary arteries. Even the once revolutionary heart transplant has become almost commonplace, with about 300 transplants carried out in the UK annually. Still more amazing possibilities lie ahead. Researchers are testing a technique that uses infrared light energy to melt away plaque in congested arteries, for instance. And there's exciting evidence that it may be possible to grow new heart muscle to replace tissue damaged during a heart attack. Eventually, researchers say, they may have the means to grow a whole new heart.

The most important advances – at least in terms of lives saved – have been in the treatment of blocked arteries. While medications that widen blood vessels and take the burden off the heart can go a long way toward relieving the symptoms of coronary artery disease, for many patients drugs aren't enough. When arteries become so obstructed that the risk of a heart attack shoots into the danger zone, doctors turn to surgical procedures. High-tech innovations are making both angioplasty and coronary bypass surgery safer and more effective than ever before. And new approaches, such as gene therapy, may one day make both of them obsolete.

Coronary bypass surgery

Coronary artery bypass grafting, as the procedure is technically known, was first performed 40 years ago. It begins with the removal of a blood vessel from a patient's leg or chest. The vessel is then reconnected near the heart in order to bypass a clogged coronary artery, creating a new channel for blood flow to the heart. When more than one vessel is obstructed, multiple grafts can be attached. The vessels that surgeons use for grafting are veins that

> High-tech innovations are making both angioplasty and coronary bypass surgery safer and more effective than ever before.

Hot topic: To stop or not to stop the heart?

Increasingly, doctors are performing bypass operations 'off pump'. Instead of using a heart-lung machine, or pump, to stop the heart, they operate while the heart is still beating. First, medications are used to slow the heart rate. Then special clamps are used to hold blood vessels still, even while blood is moving through, allowing surgeons to operate on them. In some cases, blood flow to specific blood vessels can be shut off briefly.

Some surgeons prefer off-pump bypass surgery because they believe it lowers the risks associated with stopping a patient's heart and using a heart-lung machine. (There's some evidence that being on a heart-lung machine can cause the loss of a small number of brain cells, but most doctors say the danger is minimal.) However, the procedure remains controversial. Critics worry that the advantages of off-pump surgery are outweighed by the fact that surgeons have to work faster and, because the heart is still beating, don't have as much flexibility to move vessels and manipulate the heart in order to reach obstructed arteries. Especially when several bypasses must be performed, they say, the traditional bypass is still the best bet.

FAST FACT
According to a study by the Bristol Heart Institute, off-pump surgery on over-weight people can significantly reduce deaths, shorten the amount of time spent in intensive care, cut the need for transfusions and also reduce the risk of stroke.

aren't essential to normal blood flow – which is why they can be removed and rerouted without causing blood loss elsewhere. The benefits of using a patient's own blood vessel and not a transplant or an artificial one are twofold: first, the body won't reject it, as it would a transplanted blood vessel and, second, living vessels are able to respond to blood flow by expanding or contracting as necessary – something artificial vessels couldn't do.

A commonly used vein for bypass surgery is the saphenous vein, in the leg, which is the same one that is sometimes stripped out to treat varicose veins. But surgeons have recently had considerable success in rerouting the internal mammary artery that normally supplies the chest with blood so that it feeds the heart instead. Research has demonstrated that this graft is more durable than using veins from the leg, and its use is now considered almost routine practice.

Forty years after it was first pioneered, coronary artery bypass grafting is still widely performed today. And thanks to many refinements over the years, this remarkable surgery now boasts a 98 per cent success rate. That's not bad for an operation that requires surgeons to open up the chest by splitting the sternum (breastbone) down the middle, shut down the heart and turn its function over to a heart-lung machine, and then rearrange the circulatory system.

Bypass surgery isn't a cure for heart disease, although it does help patients with severe coronary artery disease to stay alive. By letting more blood reach the heart, it cuts the risk of heart attack in half. It is also remarkably effective for easing severe angina. Eighty per cent of patients who undergo the procedure remain free of the crushing chest pain associated with coronary artery disease for at least five years.

Better bypasses

Researchers continue to devise ingenious ways to make bypass surgery even safer and more effective. One involves how surgeons connect grafted blood vessels. Traditionally, they have sewn the vessels into place with sutures. Two new techniques are faster and simpler. One uses stainless-steel clips with tiny hooks that grab onto the artery where the graft is connected. Another uses an adhesive material to connect and seal blood vessels.

Speed is the key advantage. A skilled surgeon can take up to 7 minutes to stitch one end of a vessel into place. The sutureless techniques take less than 2 minutes. Saving 5 minutes may not sound like a lot, but in operations that require many of these connections, those minutes add up – and the less time patients have to be on heart-lung machines, the less danger to the heart.

Another major advance is the development of less invasive bypass surgeries. In traditional bypasses, surgeons crack the sternum and fold back the rib cage to get to the heart. A new variation, called minimally invasive direct coronary artery bypass, or MIDCAB, allows surgeons access by way of strategically placed incisions. Part of a rib is sometimes removed to provide a window to the heart.

MIDCAB isn't for everyone. Only about 10 per cent of bypass patients qualify. The

Heart specialists usually turn to surgery when:

- ✔ Patients experience angina even when sitting still
- ✔ Drugs aren't enough to ease angina
- ✔ Angina attacks last 20 minutes or more
- ✔ The risk of a heart attack is high
- ✔ Arteries are almost completely blocked
- ✔ More than three coronary arteries are affected

▼ Key finding

Being ill can make almost anyone feel down. But undergoing heart bypass surgery may be particularly hard on your mental health, doctors are discovering. In one recent study, 65 per cent of bypass patients were depressed three weeks after surgery and 26 per cent remained depressed 12 weeks later. Researchers speculate that the unique nature of traditional bypass operations, which require stopping the heart and putting patients on heart-lung machines, may be more traumatic emotionally than other kinds of surgery. Researchers are just beginning to look into ways to ease the depression that often follows bypass surgery. The best antidote, many suspect, is to encourage patients to become physically active as soon as possible after the operation.

Is surgery really necessary?

Surprisingly, choosing between medication and surgery isn't always easy. Thanks to recent advances, both approaches are yielding better outcomes. For some patients, in fact, they may be equally effective.

Researchers at Washington University analysed results from more than a dozen separate clinical trials involving thousands of patients treated for coronary artery disease. They found that 90 per cent of patients who were given drugs to help to keep blood flowing to their hearts were still alive five years later compared with 94 per cent of patients who underwent heart bypass surgery. Bypasses were initially more effective at relieving angina. But after five years, the patients on drug therapy experienced just as much relief.

In some instances drugs can actually be more effective than surgery. In 1999 *The New England Journal of Medicine* reported surprising results from a study of 341 patients who were suffering from coronary artery disease but were experiencing only mild to moderate angina. Half were randomly chosen to receive a cholesterol-lowering drug; the others underwent angioplasty.

Eighteen months later only 22 per cent of those taking the medication had experienced chest pain compared with 37 per cent of the angioplasty patients.

How do doctors decide which path to take? The severity of symptoms is one factor. If you have unstable angina – chest pain that occurs even when you aren't exerting yourself – or your angina attacks last for 20 minutes or more, you may be a candidate for surgery. And if you've been on medications, but they aren't doing enough to relieve angina, surgery may be the next step. The extent of the blockages in your coronary arteries is another consideration.

Age also comes into it – patients aged 75 or older seem to fare better with bypass surgery than medication. In one recent study half of those on medication had experienced a heart attack or other coronary event compared with only 19 per cent of those who had received bypasses or angioplasties.

Of course the choice isn't one or the other. Anyone who is treated for angina or coronary artery disease will have to have a number of medications, lifelong, irrespective of whether they also undergo surgery or angioplasty.

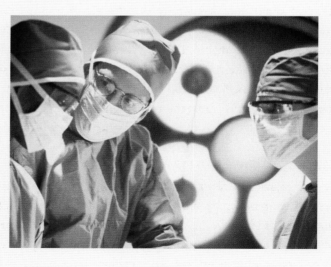

reason: the procedure is most effective when used to bypass clogged arteries at the front of the heart, which are readily accessible through a small incision.

Growing new blood vessels

Researchers may soon have a bold new way to give traditional bypasses a boost. In research funded by the National Heart, Lung, and Blood Institute, Harvard scientists inserted timed-release capsules containing a substance that promotes the growth of new blood vessels into the heart muscle of patients scheduled for bypass surgery. Patients in a second group were given a placebo substance. Tests showed that those who received the active substance, called basic fibroblast growth factor, had better blood flow into their heart muscles than those who were given the placebo. They were also less likely to suffer angina after surgery. By spurring the growth of small blood vessels, researchers believe, growth factors ensure that blood from the grafted artery reaches more parts of the heart.

Indeed, growth factors like these may eventually offer an alternative to surgery. In 2001 researchers injected the gene for a growth-promoting substance called vascular endothelial growth factor, or VEGF, directly into the hearts of patients with advanced coronary artery disease who were too sick to undergo surgery. The gene stimulates the production of a naturally occurring protein involved in growing new blood vessels. In one study using VEGF, a majority of patients reported less angina and greater mobility after the treatment. In another study involving 30 patients, 27 reported fewer angina attacks and said they took less nitroglycerin after the treatment.

For now VEGF remains experimental. The British Heart Foundation recently reported that trials for patients with heart failure might soon be underway. And if those studies confirm its effectiveness and safety, VEGF could become one of the first approved uses of gene therapy to treat heart disease.

Angioplasty as an alternative

In recent years cardiologists have increasingly turned to a less invasive way to resupply blood to the heart: a technique called angioplasty (its full name is percutaneous transluminal coronary angioplasty). Instead of bypassing blocked coronary arteries, doctors reopen obstructed vessels, allowing more blood to flow through them. Angioplasty is especially useful for relieving angina.

FAST FACT

In the UK, the number of coronary bypass operations has almost doubled in 10 years – in 2000–2001 doctors performed 28,500 operations, compared with 16,000 in 1990.

| Hot topic: | Angioplasty or bypass surgery? |

If your angiogram shows that your angina is caused by one or more blockages or narrowings in the coronary arteries, your specialist will decide whether your arteries can be improved by angioplasty or whether surgery is the best option. You may be suitable for either, in which case you will be offered a choice. There are advantages and disadvantages to both. With angioplasty, you are more likely to get angina again, and may end up having to have surgery in the future. Other considerations when comparing angioplasty and surgery are:

- You will have a local anaesthetic as opposed to a general anaesthetic
- Your hospital stay is 1 or 2 days, compared with 6 to 10 days
- You can return to work after 5 to 7 days, compared with 2 to 3 months
- Three in every 100 people need angioplasty again within 6 months, compared with 1 or 2 in a 100 needing further surgery
- Five in every 1000 people die within 30 days of the angioplasty, compared with 20 in every 1000 who have surgery.

It involves threading a flexible tube called a catheter, about the diameter of a pencil, through a small incision, usually made in the groin or the arm, and into a main artery. The catheter is then guided into the coronary arteries. Radio-opaque dye – visible under X-ray – is injected so that cardiologists can view the area around the heart and find the exact location of the obstruction. Then they can clear away the blockage and reopen the clogged blood vessel.

The most common technique uses a catheter with a tiny balloon attached to its tip. Once the tip reaches the obstruction, the balloon is inflated and deflated several times, compressing the fatty deposits in the artery against the vessel wall and so reopening the channel. Another, less common technique, called an atherectomy, uses a catheter tipped with a miniature cutting tool, like a dentist's drill, to file away the cholesterol-laden plug blocking blood flow.

Risks and benefits
By letting more blood reach the heart, angioplasty greatly reduces symptoms of angina and cuts the risk of a heart attack. But there is some risk that the procedure may trigger a heart attack. As cholesterol-laden plaque is broken down during the operation, tiny pieces may break loose and be carried into smaller arteries, creating a jam, known as an embolism, and blocking blood flow.

The risk of a heart attack triggered by angioplasty is generally about 5 per cent. But the danger can jump as high as 15 per cent in patients who have bypass grafts or stents in place. However, new

REAL PEOPLE, REAL WISDOM

Listen to your body

In 2003, after running the London Marathon and another long-distance race in Bournemouth, Iain Price, 54, decided to give his body a well-earned rest.

He took a month off, but when he started running again, it just didn't feel right. His usual lunchtime runs or his early morning runs from the New Forest to work on the coast, were feeling really tough.

'I could only run for five miles,' says Iain. 'I felt generally run down and thought I had a virus that I just couldn't shake off. Also, I had indigestion a couple of times, but didn't think much of it – the pain was soon gone.'

His colleagues at work finally persuaded him to see his doctor, who performed an ECG and told him that he had an unusual heart-beat and needed to see a specialist.

Iain wasn't worried. He knew that his cholesterol was a bit high, and his job involved long hours and some stress, but he was fit and didn't eat to excess. Although both his father and his brother had suffered heart disease, Iain didn't make the connection.

In December, he went for his first ever hospital appointment and had another ECG, a cholesterol test and a treadmill test. The cardiologist then told him that he would carry out an angiogram. It came as quite a surprise when Iain was told that he needed a triple heart bypass. He was also told to take time off work straight away.

In January 2004, Iain had his bypass surgery. 'While I was sitting there in the hospital, waiting for surgery, I felt a bit of a fraud – I still didn't feel there was anything wrong with me', says Iain.

The operation was a success and his doctors are pleased with his recovery. He takes statins now, and his cholesterol level has dropped dramatically. The Bournemouth Heart Hospital offered a seven-week cardiac rehabilitation programme that helped him to get back his strength.

'I found it quite easy, because I was fit before the surgery, but it was a great way to get back into shape. The physiotherapists there tell you what you can and cannot do, and that's reassuring. The Heart Club not only advised him on his exercise routines, but also gave him detailed information on what foods to eat and what to avoid.

'The chips are gone', says Iain ruefully 'but I've discovered roasted vegetables and there are some delicious fat-free foods out there – it's opened up a new world of food for me.'

Iain is already looking for new challenges. He did the Great South Run on October 10th, 2004, less than nine months after his surgery – and is now training for a half marathon. And who knows? A full marathon in 2006?

'Here I am now – a man who's had a triple bypass,' says Iain. 'I feel as well as before; the only thing I have is a couple of scars.'

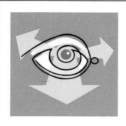

LOOKING AHEAD
Melting plaques with light

Even in the most skilled hands, catheters used during angioplasty can damage artery walls, making the arteries more vulnerable to new blockages. A more subtle approach to clearing away coronary artery obstructions could solve the problem. It is an experimental technique called photoangioplasty, and surgeons use infrared light to melt away plaques without touching healthy artery cells around them.

First, they inject a light-sensitive chemical that is absorbed by the plaque but not the surrounding cells. Then a very narrow catheter is guided to the site, where it emits high-frequency light energy. This energy stimulates the light-sensitive chemical, which in turn destroys the obstruction, leaving healthy cells undisturbed. Although photoangioplasty is still in the early stages of testing, many researchers think it will offer an effective alternative to standard angioplasty in coming years.

gadgets (embolization protection devices) promise to lower the risk dramatically. The new devices are really nothing more than tiny filters, about the size of a pencil eraser. They are threaded into position down-stream from the artery blockage, where they catch up to 93 per cent of the debris that breaks loose.

There is another serious problem associated with angioplasties that has not been as easy to solve. In one out of three patients, blockages re-form in coronary arteries within three to six months after the procedure, a phenomenon called restenosis. The new blockages aren't the same as the cholesterol-laden plaques that cause coronary artery disease in the first place. Small blood clots and the build-up of cholesterol may play a role; but damage can be inflicted on the lining of blood vessels during angioplasty. When the lining is disturbed, immune cells rush in to repair the damage, triggering the growth of new cells. These new cells form thickened patches, which in turn reduce blood flow through the artery.

Exactly why some patients suffer restenosis and other don't is still something of a mystery. In a study reported in 2001, researchers from New Zealand followed 2,690 angioplasty patients. Six months after surgery, angiograms showed that 607 of them had developed new blockages. Half of them had no angina symptoms to alert doctors to the problem. Men were more likely than women to have so-called 'silent' restenosis, but the researchers found nothing else in the patients' medical histories that would predict who developed restenosis.

When new blockages form, surgeons often have to perform another angioplasty. If blockages recur, bypass surgery may be necessary. Now, however, there's exciting evidence that scientists may have finally put the problem of reblockage to rest.

Block that blockage

The first giant step in preventing restenosis came with the introduction of devices called stents, expandable metal-mesh tubes implanted after an artery is widened in order to keep the channel open. Stents are now implanted in about 95 per cent of all angioplasty patients. These simple devices have proved so successful that more and more surgeons are skipping the balloon entirely and simply using a stent to open clogged arteries. Researchers recently reported that this 'direct stenting' is just as effective as implanting a stent after balloon angioplasty. And it offers two distinct advantages: shorter operating time and lower costs.

The use of stents has cut the danger of new blockages from about 40 per cent to only 15 to 20 per cent. And another approach, called coronary brachytherapy, is lowering the risk even further. Surgeons expose the lining of newly unclogged arteries to a small dose of radiation, which has been shown to reduce the occurrence of new obstructions by approximately 60 per cent.

The most significant advance in treating patients with angina, and reducing the rate of restenosis after angioplasty and stent insertion is the use of drug-eluting coronary stents. These are

FAST FACT
The number of angioplasties performed in the UK has quadrupled in ten years: more than 45,000 were performed in 2002.

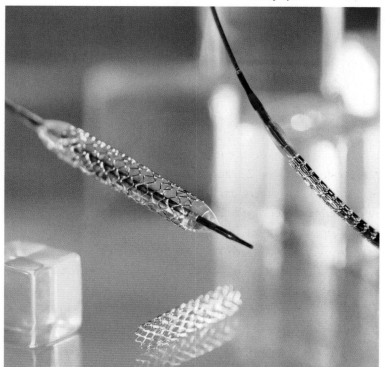

After angioplasty, a small metal tube called a stent may be inserted to keep the artery open.

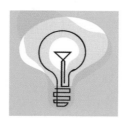

ASK THE EXPERT

With advances coming along so quickly, how can I make sure my doctor is taking advantage of the latest breakthroughs?

Dr Stanley Rockson, associate professor of cardiovascular medicine at Stanford University:

'It's easy to get caught up in all the excitement surrounding the state-of-the-art techniques making headlines. But it's important to put these new discoveries in perspective. One of the great strengths of the medical system is the push to innovate – to find new and better ways to treat illnesses and help people to stay well. But another strength is caution. We insist that new drugs or surgical techniques be carefully tested and the results documented so doctors know what works and what doesn't.

And believe me, there are plenty of examples of promising new ideas that didn't pan out quite the way we expected them to. Take laser angioplasty, for instance. For a time, all of us in the field were very excited about the prospect of using lasers to burn away plaque on the inside of arteries. Mostly we hoped the technique would help prevent restenosis. Hospitals around the country bought hundreds of fancy laser-based angioplasty devices. Unfortunately, laser angioplasty didn't turn out to be any better than the traditional approach, and many of those devices now sit in hospital corridors covered with sheets. Right now there is interest in another new approach, called photoangioplasty, which uses a light-sensitive chemical and infrared light to remove plaque. Only time, and thorough testing, will tell if it is a bona fide advance.

Indeed, it takes three to five years to test a new approach to find out whether it's truly safe and effective – and once something is approved, it takes another three to five years for doctors using it in their practices to decide whether it really is any better than traditional approaches.

For 95 per cent or more of patients with coronary artery disease, the best chance of success is tried-and-trusted treatments with proven value. Certainly if you've read about something that sounds exciting, ask your doctor. But remember, you're usually better off in the hands of a surgeon who is using a technique he or she trusts and has done many times before than with some new and unproven approach.'

stents coated with a polymer that is impregnated with a substance that is released slowly from the stent and prevents the restenosis process almost completely. Cardiologists in the UK are now treating twice as many people with this technology than they are with traditional coronary artery bypass surgery.

Which surgery to choose?

How do doctors decide when to perform bypass surgery and when to use angioplasty? The decision typically involves weighing many factors. One important advantage of angioplasty is the fact that it is far less invasive. But it usually isn't as effective in resupplying blood to the heart, especially over the long haul. So doctors often perform angioplasty first, hoping that it will do the trick. If it doesn't, they may turn to bypass surgery.

Sometimes, however, angioplasties aren't practical – if too many arteries are blocked, for example, or one artery is obstructed with a blockage so large that the artery can't be opened by a catheter. Surgeons used to avoid angioplasty for patients with diabetes, because the disease causes damage to blood vessels, and the trauma of inserting a catheter could cause further damage. But with the advent of drug-eluting stents, they can now treat a wider range of patients, including diabetics.

Of course bypasses aren't always practical – when patients are too frail to withstand the operation, for instance. Or when previous bypasses have been performed and there are no more blood vessels left to graft.

New approaches, new hope

When drugs aren't powerful enough, and bypasses or angioplasties aren't practical, there's still hope. Doctors have been experimenting with a technique called transmyocardial revascularization, or TMR, which involves drilling tiny holes into heart muscle. No one really knows why the technique works, although the holes do seem to allow more blood to reach heart muscle cells. Several studies have shown that TMR can bring relief to people with angina. Because the holes eventually heal over, however, the benefits are usually short-lived.

Surprisingly successful for many patients is a technique that has been imported from China, called enhanced external counter-pulsation, or EECP. To look at it, you wouldn't think EECP had anything to do with the heart. Pressurized cuffs are placed around a patient's upper and lower legs. Then an air pump inflates and deflates the cuffs, squeezing leg muscles and forcing blood up into the heart. The pump is precisely synchronized to inflate the cuffs each time the heart relaxes between beats, producing a 'counter-pulse' that creates additional blood pressure when blood is refilling the heart's chambers.

Questions to ask when you face surgery

✔ How is the operation done?
✔ What is the purpose of the operation?
✔ Are there alternatives to surgery?
✔ What will you gain by having the operation?
✔ What are the possible complications and side effects?
✔ Why should the operation be done now?
✔ How often has the surgeon performed this operation?
✔ What is the surgeon's success rate?
✔ What complications has he or she encountered?
✔ How will you feel after the surgery?
✔ How long will your recovery take?
✔ Is there anything you can do to speed your recovery?

Again, scientists aren't exactly sure why counterpulsation seems to ease angina. The technique has been shown to widen arteries that feed the heart, especially smaller arteries that don't normally play a big role in supplying blood to heart muscles. EECP also appears to spur the growth of new coronary arteries.

Whatever the reason, it seems to work. In a study at the State University of New York at Stony Brook, researchers tested EECP in 18 patients with advanced coronary artery disease. The hour-long procedure was repeated 35 times over seven weeks. All 18 patients reported much less angina. Sixteen were completely free of chest pain during their normal activities. Imaging tests showed that artery blockages were reduced in 14 of the 18 patients.

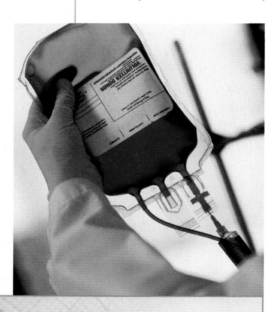

At present, doctors perform EECP only when other, more traditional approaches fail. It is available at a few NHS centres but otherwise only privately – a full course may cost as much as £10,500. Some researchers think that the technique should play a role in treating patients newly diagnosed with coronary artery disease. By stimulating increased blood flow to the heart, EECP could help prevent angina and ward off heart attacks, they say.

▼ Key finding

A simple blood transfusion can make a big difference to the chances of survival of patients with heart failure, according to a 2001 Yale University study. Examining records from 78,974 elderly people, researchers found that 40 per cent were anaemic. Those with the lowest red blood cell counts were twice as likely as those with normal blood readings to die during the first month after a heart attack. What makes this finding specially worrying is that only a quarter of the anaemic patients studied were given blood transfusions to boost their red blood cell levels. Patients who did receive blood transfusions dramatically improved their odds of surviving a heart attack. By publishing their results, the Yale team hopes to encourage doctors to test more patients for anaemia – and to offer those with low red blood cell counts potentially lifesaving transfusions.

New help for failing hearts

Coronary artery disease, severe high blood pressure, heart attacks – all three can leave the heart too weak to supply

ASK THE EXPERT

Is it normal to feel anxious or depressed after heart surgery – and is there anything I can do?

Helen Booth RGN BSc, Nurse Practitioner at the Holborn Medical Centre in London:

'Of course there is. Many people who've had a heart attack or undergone cardiac surgery feel anxious or depressed afterwards. The experience can be very frightening. Once you have been discharged from hospital, you are not under the surveillance of doctors and nurses. It's natural to wonder if your heart is going to keep working as it did and whether you'll be able to make the lifestyle changes you need to keep you healthy.

Being alert to how you feel is important to your recovery. Research has shown that anxiety or depression slow your recovery. Stress puts a strain on your heart, increases blood pressure, and can even affect cholesterol levels.

Stress shows itself in three different ways. Physiological symptoms include muscle tension, racing heart, excess sweating, trembling and stomach complaints. Behavioural symptoms may affect your sleeping pattern; you may not sleep as well as usual, or you wake very early and can't go back to sleep. Or you may stop getting pleasure out of things you used to love, or feel huge frustration at the smallest things. Finally, there are cognitive symptoms – memory loss, poor concentration and mental confusion.

Many cardiac rehabilitation programmes focus on four main strategies to help heart patients to relieve stress and ease depression.

The first is learning relaxation techniques – deep-breathing exercises that help you to focus your thoughts and relax your muscles. The second strategy is exercise. Physical activities like walking are a great way to manage stress and also to get the added heart benefits of exercise. Third, you should be encouraged to try to connect with friends and family. Studies show that people who are isolated are more likely to get sick and relapse than people with a strong social network. So now is the time to get more involved. Look for activities in your community. Or simply phone some old friends and catch up.

Finally, it's important to do things you enjoy. That may sound like common sense. But when people are feeling depressed, they tend to become reclusive. On the other hand, when people pursue pleasurable activities – when they push themselves to get out and go for a walk in a favourite park, visit a friend or see a play or attend a concert – they get themselves out of a rut and start feeling better about their lives.

There's another benefit to getting up and doing something. The more you do, the more confident you'll feel about your health. That confidence will help you to stay motivated to make the changes necessary to live a heart healthy lifestyle.'

enough blood to meet the body's needs. An estimated 878,000 people in Britain suffer from heart failure and 63,000 new cases are diagnosed each year. Heart medications have made a big difference for many of them. But drugs aren't always powerful enough to ease the burden on failing hearts, and doctors have to turn to surgery.

The potential of mechanical pumps

The human heart is a pump – nothing more and nothing less. When hearts fail, the problem usually lies with the left ventricle, the chamber that pumps blood to the entire body. Miniaturized pumps, called ventricular assist devices, can be implanted in the chest to help to push blood forward. The newest versions work like tiny jet engines, moving blood at a steady pace. As a result, patients no

Keeping the pace

In as many as half the people with heart failure, the left and right ventricles, the heart's main pumping chambers, don't contract at exactly the same time; as a result the heart becomes less efficient at pumping out blood to the rest of the body. A new type of pacemaker, invented in the USA and approved for use in the UK in 2002, synchronizes the two chambers, boosting the heart's pumping power and improving the quality of life of the people who receive it. The device allows patients to be more active, less out of breath, and less tired.

Pacemakers are small implantable devices that deliver electrical charges to keep the heart beating regularly. Most are used to treat heartbeat irregularities, or arrhythmias. Traditional pacemakers commonly supply two wires to the heart: one to the upper right chamber (the right atrium) and one to the lower right chamber (the right ventricle). The InSync Biventricular Cardiac Pacing System has a third wire that connects to the lower left chamber, synchronizing the two ventricles. Like other high-tech pacemakers, the InSync even slows down or speeds up according to the person's activity level.

To test the InSync device, researchers implanted the pacemaker (about the size of a small coin) in 532 patients with heart failure but only turned it on in 263 of them. During the next three to six months, the people with the activated pacemaker were able to walk farther and scored higher on a test that measures quality of life. At the end of the study, the researchers turned on the pacemakers in the other patients so that they could benefit from it too.

longer have a normal heartbeat. This lack of a pulse makes it difficult for doctors to measure a patient's blood pressure, since blood pressure gauges depend on counting heartbeats. But even this problem is being solved. The latest pumps can check on conditions in the body and transmit data to doctors to help them to monitor their patients.

Traditionally, mechanical pumps have been thought of as a 'bridge' treatment – a way to keep patients with serious heart failure alive while they waited for heart transplants. Because donor hearts are so scarce, however, many patients have ended up on these pumps for extended periods of time – in some cases up to four years. So doctors began to wonder whether the pumps themselves might offer a permanent alternative to heart transplantation. To find out more, the Columbia University College of Physicians and Surgeons in Manhattan enlisted 129 patients with heart failure who were not eligible for transplants because they were either too sick or too old. Some of the volunteers were then given a mechanical pump called the HeartMate, which is implanted in the abdomen. The rest of the volunteers were treated with drugs known to help to ease the burden on failing hearts.

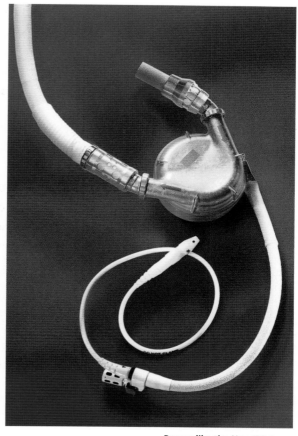

Pumps like the HeartMate can help people with serious heart failure to live longer.

The HeartMate uses one tube to drain blood from the left ventricle into the mechanical pump. Another tube pumps it back into the aorta, from which it flows out to the body. A third passes through the skin to an external battery pack and control system. The Columbia study proved that these little pumps are lifesavers. A year after they were installed 52 per cent of patients were still alive – compared with only 25 per cent of those who received the best available drug treatments. After two years 23 per cent of patients with the pumps were still alive compared with only 8 per cent of those on medications.

Cardiothoracic surgeon Steven Westaby from John Radcliffe, Oxford, says mechanical pumps could prevent some 20,000 deaths from heart failure in the UK every year. At present, however, this

Emergency help when you need it

An estimated 27,000 people in the UK die each year of cardiac arrest, which is often caused by ventricular fibrillation – when the lower chambers of the heart rapidly contract out of sync. A defibrillator that delivers a jolt of electricity to shock the heart back into beating normally could save many of those lives, but only if one is available. Too often it isn't. But there is now a new defibrillator that can be worn on the body.

The device, called LifeVest, contains four sensors, strapped to the chest, that

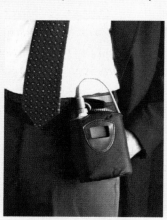

monitor heartbeat. When they notice an irregular heart rhythm, they signal a miniature defibrillator, worn on a belt around the waist, to deliver a shock to the heart.

In a study of 289 patients the device was successful 71 per cent of the time in detecting and treating sudden cardiac arrest compared with a success rate of only 25 per cent when people call 999. Experts say the device will be useful for people following a serious heart attack and for patients awaiting a heart transplant.

technique is not funded by the NHS, so it is very expensive. There is government approval for 12 Jarvik pumps (similar to the US HeartMate and named after its UK inventor) to be implanted experimentally; however, the work must be funded privately. A new miniature Jarvik 2000 Heart, which fits within the patient's own failing heart, is currently undergoing trials.

The gift of life

The very idea of transplanting a living heart from one person to another still seems miraculous, but about 300 heart transplants are performed in the UK each year. Researchers have made giant strides in controlling the biggest problem of transplantation: rejection of the transplanted organ. New drugs effectively suppress the body's immune system so it won't attack the new organ, allowing the transplanted heart to go on beating.

The biggest limitation is a lack of donor hearts. At any given time in the UK about 120 people are waiting for a new heart, but there are not enough donors and 15 in every 100 patients die while on the waiting list. Efforts are underway to improve the organ donor information network so that more hearts and other organs become available. Still, the transplantation of living hearts will never offer a complete solution to the problem of heart failure. As an alternative, researchers have dreamed for years of creating a mechanical organ that would beat as reliably as our own heart. Recently that dream became reality.

The bionic heart – a new solution?

In July 2001 the world's first truly bionic heart began beating – or rather clicking – in the chest of a human patient. The man who made medical history was a retired telephone company employee named Robert Tools, whose own heart was failing rapidly. As he told reporters at Jewish Hospital in Louisville, Kentucky, where the operation was performed, 'I had a choice to sit at home and die or come in here and take a chance'.

That chance paid off. The 3lb (1.35kg) artificial heart implanted in his chest kept him alive for 151 days. It was an engineering marvel. In the past, artificial hearts had to be connected by wires that passed through the skin to a power supply unit, creating a constant risk of serious infection. The newest artificial heart, called the AbioCor, is equipped with its own rechargeable battery that allows the device to be fully self-contained. Most of the time, a small battery pack worn outside the body sends radio waves to power the AbioCor. But the rechargeable battery can also run on its own for up to 45 minutes, allowing patients to bathe or go swimming, for instance. A microchip in the heart allows it to adjust its rate to what patients are doing.

These devices are not used in the UK, and experts believe that assisting rather than replacing a failing heart is preferable. A bionic heart is prone to mechanical failure, which means instant death. Also, the bionic heart has a large surface area that could attract infection, and it carries a great risk of bursting delicate haemoglobin red cells. Steven Westaby, at Oxford's John Radcliffe Hospital, favours replacing the heart with two small pumps instead of one. This gives the heart a chance to rest and recover.

The AbioCor is the first artificial heart to be fully enclosed inside the body.

More achievements ahead

It's remarkable enough that surgeons have learned how to transplant living hearts and construct an entirely artificial one. But what if researchers could discover a way in which to encourage damaged hearts to heal themselves? What if they could trigger the body to grow new heart muscle – or even a whole new heart?

Such hopes were the stuff of science fiction until recently. Now several studies offer encouraging evidence that heart muscle can be regenerated and, possibly, new hearts grown.

Researchers have known for years that the bone marrow, the liver and the lining of the intestines can regenerate, replacing damaged or diseased tissue with new healthy cells. But most experts assumed that the heart lacked the ability to grow new cells.

Then, in 2001, investigators in New York discovered something startling: what looked like brand-new heart muscle cells in areas near where a heart attack had occurred. At the time, the scientists didn't know whether these were simply existing heart cells that had divided to form new cells or entirely new cells, born of stem cells, which are the progenitors of all the specialized tissues in the body.

Now they know, thanks to a experiment reported in *The New England Journal of Medicine* in January 2002. The New York team transplanted eight hearts from female donors into male patients. When the team looked at new heart muscle cells that had developed, they found that 10 per cent of them contained a Y chromosome, the definitive marker of a male cell. The evidence proved that stem cells from

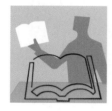

TERMS TO KNOW

ANGIOPLASTY A procedure in which a narrow tube called a catheter is threaded into blocked coronary arteries in order to clear an obstruction, often using a tiny balloon that's inflated and deflated several times to reopen the vessel

CORONARY ARTERY BYPASS GRAFTING An operation that involves removing a blood vessel from the leg or other part of the body and grafting it near the heart to bypass a clogged coronary artery

EMBOLISM A blood clot that forms in a blood vessel in one part of the body and travels to another part

PACEMAKER A miniature electronic device implanted in the chest and wired to the heart to control the heartbeat

RESTENOSIS The formation of new blockages after either angioplasty or bypass surgery has been performed

STEM CELLS Primitive cells created in the bone marrow that can develop into any of the many specialized cells of the body

STENT An expandable metal-mesh tube that is placed inside an obstructed artery to widen the vessel and keep it open

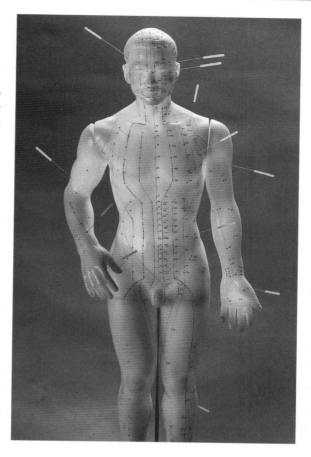

Acupuncture points on different parts of the body relate to pain in specific organs and areas.

the patients had migrated into the heart and were helping to replace muscle cells injured during the transplant operation.

This extraordinary finding raises hopes that scientists may eventually be able to harness the power of stem cells, encouraging the heart to repair itself after a heart attack or other injury. Indeed, some scientists have already tried to do exactly that. In a study that was reported in 2002, a French doctor implanted stem cells from a heart patient's thigh muscle into his ailing heart. The cells developed into healthy heart muscle cells and strengthened the heart.

The British Heart Foundation has funded research into which type of bone marrow stem cells will restore heart function in the long term. The debate on stem cell research has a long way to go, but hope exists for great achievements.

▼ Key finding

One of the world's oldest healing techniques may help people with severe heart failure, according to results reported at the American Heart Association's 2001 conference. Acupuncture, the practice of inserting needles into the skin at specific points, was shown to ease the burden on ailing hearts by reducing sympathetic nerve activity. (The sympathetic nervous system, or 'emergency response system', is charged with increasing heart rate and blood pressure and rushing blood into the muscles as part of the 'fight or flight' response.) That's important, because heart failure patients have two to three times more sympathetic nerve activity than healthy people. The greater that activity, the worse the prognosis. Further studies are needed to confirm the new promise of this ancient technique.

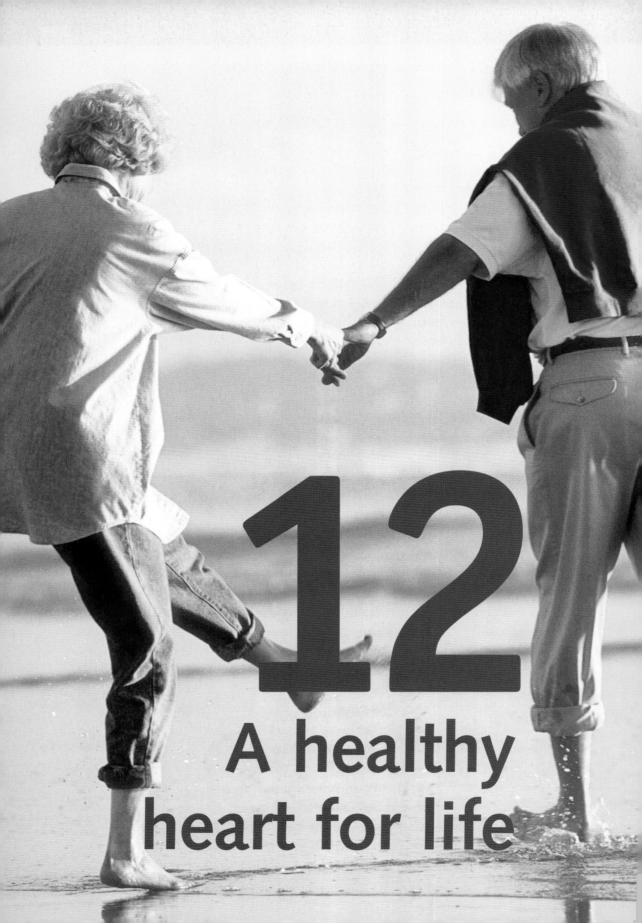

12
A healthy heart for life

There's no doubt that cardiologists today can work wonders for the heart, but the most powerful medicine is still what you do for yourself. That's true even after you've suffered a heart attack or undergone heart surgery. The same steps that can help to prevent heart disease in the first place – from eating more sensibly to being more active – will speed your recovery and dramatically reduce your odds of further trouble.

It really is never too late to start taking care of your heart. If you're a smoker who's had a heart attack, for instance, you can cut your risk of having another in half by kicking the habit now. If you've been diagnosed with coronary artery disease, lifestyle changes can halt and perhaps even reverse the process of atherosclerosis, opening up clogged arteries. There's another benefit, too: starting healthy new habits can help you to regain a feeling of control over your health and feel more positive about the future.

Lifestyle plays such a powerful role in helping heart patients recover after a heart attack or surgery that many hospitals now offer formal cardiac rehabilitation programmes. Most focus on that vital threesome: exercise, diet and stress reduction. The real benefit is the close supervision and encouragement they offer, as well as the support of other patients in the same situation. Several studies have shown that people who enroll in cardiac rehabilitation get better and become active sooner than those who don't. However, only a third of patients discharged after a heart attack are receiving cardiac rehabilitation, which is well below the government's target of 85 per cent. If a rehabilitation programme is not available to you, don't despair. With your doctor's help and advice, you can create your own programme for recovery.

If you've been diagnosed with coronary artery disease, lifestyle changes can halt and perhaps even reverse the process of atherosclerosis, opening up clogged arteries.

On the road to recovery

The first thing to focus on is becoming physically active again. There was a time when cardiologists advised patients to take it easy, even to remain in bed for weeks after a heart attack or surgery. Not any more. The sooner you get up and get moving, experts now say, the faster you'll recover – even if you've had very serious heart problems. According to the British Heart Foundation, physical activity has been shown to be helpful in the period after a heart attack and reduces the risk of dying by 20 per cent. If you were a couch potato before your attack, you will probably be advised to gradually become more active; if you were quite fit, your goal will be to resume your former exercise habits.

How much you can safely do is for your cardiologist to say. Most rehabilitation programmes encourage people to begin slowly and gradually add more – and more strenuous – activities, beginning with walking and progressing to pedalling on an exercise bike, jogging, swimming or other activities. How hard you should push yourself depends on what you've just been through, how active you were in the past, and your overall health. Your ultimate goal should be at least 30 minutes of moderately intense exercise – a brisk walk or the equivalent – most days of the week.

If you experience chest pain while exercising, tell your doctor. Discuss any worries you have about physical activity, but don't let fear stop you from reaping the benefits of exercise. In a study of 68 patients so sick that they were on a waiting list for heart transplants, an exercise programme alone proved so successful at easing their symptoms and improving coronary artery blood flow that 31 were healthy enough to be removed from the transplant list.

Once you're up and moving again, take a fresh look at your diet. Cut back on saturated fat; consume more fruit and vegetables; eat more whole-grain foods. But there's new urgency if you have been diagnosed with heart disease. One of the major benefits of a heart-healthy diet is its effect on LDL cholesterol, the artery-clogging kind. And if you have coronary artery disease, you need to try to get your LDL level down even further than people whose arteries are clear. According to experts, people with no risk factor or one risk factor can get away with an LDL level under 4.1mmol/l. People with two or more risk factors should strive to get theirs below 3.3mmol/l. But if you have heart disease, your ideal LDL level is under 2.5mmol/l. Your doctor may recommend a cholesterol-lowering drug to bring your levels down, but you can help by improving your diet.

TROUBLESHOOTING TIP

Men suffering from heart failure often have trouble maintaining erections because their hearts can't pump enough blood throughout the body. Exercise can help, according to a study by experts at the Lancisi Heart Institute in Italy. Among a group of 59 men with heart failure, those who cycled 40 minutes three times a week for eight weeks dramatically improved their scores on a standard questionnaire used to gauge sexual function. They also improved their overall quality of life.

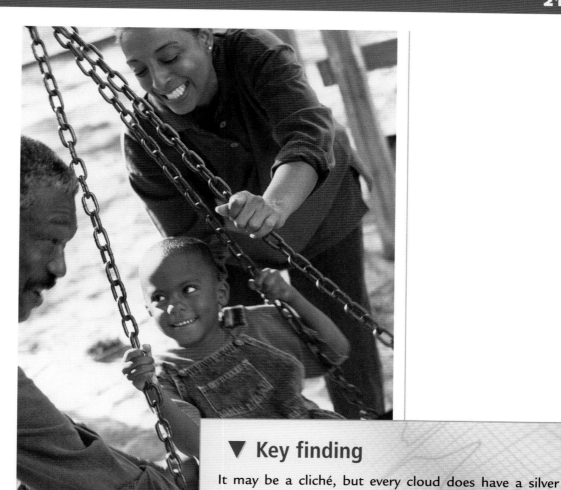

▼ Key finding

It may be a cliché, but every cloud does have a silver lining. In a recent survey, one out of three patients reported that their quality of life had actually improved after suffering a heart attack. Patients reported an increased joy in being alive, closer relationships with their loved ones, a clearer grasp of what really matters in their lives and a sense of well-being thanks to healthier habits.

Finally, there's the issue of stress. Finding ways to relax is a good idea no matter what your state of health, but it's even more important if you've been diagnosed with heart disease. Any serious illness creates its own stresses. It can even force difficult decisions, such as whether to keep working or retire. Unfortunately, the same emotional strain caused by heart disease can slow your recovery. In fact, a high degree of psychological stress after a heart attack has been shown to be an independent risk factor for dying within the next year.

The good news is that even in the face of something as serious as heart disease, simple relaxation techniques can make a real difference. In one study, researchers compared a group of heart patients who were given relaxation audio tapes in the cardiac care unit with patients who received standard care. The tapes contained spoken instructions for progressive muscle relaxation and deep breathing exercises. Four months later, the patients who received the tapes were walking further and suffering fewer episodes of chest pain. Just as important, half as many as those in the other group reported having emotional difficulties. You can find a variety of relaxation tapes at bookstores and online. Many hospitals offer stress reduction programmes that include both counselling and aids such as audio tapes.

REAL PEOPLE, REAL WISDOM

There is life after a heart attack

Graham Marsh, 49, from North Shields, Tyne and Wear, was a busy family man and self-employed salesman. In his spare time he was secretary of the local football team and chairman of the Tyne Boys' club.

One evening in May 1999 while he was watching football on TV Graham suddenly felt such severe chest pain that he was rolling round the floor in agony. His wife ran to fetch their neighbour, a cardiac nurse, who gave him an aspirin, which he is convinced saved his life. Within minutes he was rushed to hospital.

Graham spent only a week in hospital and seemed to be making good progress, but back home he experienced the pain again. After more tests it was decided that he needed a triple heart bypass, which in the event turned out to be a quintuple. 'But still my heart was just too weakened after the attack and when they took me off the ventilator I thought I was dying,' he says.

Doctors decided then that the only possible option was a heart transplant.

For three months after the transplant Graham was in self-imposed quarantine, taking care not to catch an infection, but gradually returned to 'normal life'. The hospital physiotherapist was a great help in getting him back in shape. 'When all I wanted to do was wallow in self pity, she'd breeze in and, before I knew it, it was down to the hospital gym.'

Graham now watches his diet, goes to the gym twice a week, plays two or three rounds of golf a week and regularly goes out for walks. 'In hospital I set myself a new goal – to run one lap of Gateshead International Stadium. The day I did it was at the 2000 British Transplant Games and I won the 100m. It was one of the proudest days of my life.'

Graham has travelled the world competing in the Transplant Games and won medals in the 100m, relays and long jump. He is now Team Manager for the Freeman Transplant Sports Team. 'Many people think heart disease is the end, but for me it was the beginning of a new way of life' he says proudly.

Meeting the challenge ahead

Remember the old bumper sticker that read 'Today is the first day of the rest of your life'? It's a cliché, but it captures an essential truth. Today really can be the beginning of a healthier life. New drugs and treatments can help. But the rest is up to you.

It will not always be easy. Even people who have been shocked into action by serious heart problems sometimes find it difficult to overcome a lifetime of unhealthy habits. They may be enthusiastic at first – or at least grimly determined. But after the first month, researchers find, people's commitment begins to fade. By the end of six months, evidence shows, too many have abandoned their best intentions.

The reason is almost certainly that, like the proverbial old dog, it's not easy for people to learn new tricks. Habits have a way of becoming deeply ingrained. And it's not just a matter of being stuck in a rut. Some habits, like smoking, are physically addictive. Others become hard-wired into our brains, much the same way a learned skill like riding a bike becomes programmed into our neural pathways. Anything we repeat again and again becomes a learned behaviour. That's fine, if all your habits are healthy ones. If they're not, breaking them can be a challenge.

But it can be done. If you get into the practice of walking around the neighbourhood instead of turning on the TV after dinner, you'll gradually find it's easier to take the pavement instead of the armchair. Make a habit of having fruit for dessert, and it won't take long before you're looking forward to the taste of a baked apple, a bowl of ripe cherries or orange and grapefruit sections splashed with liqueur. You won't erase the old habit – you'll probably still be tempted to vegetate in front of the TV after dinner, for instance. And no doubt you'll want to treat yourself to a slice of chocolate cake now and then. (And once in a while you should.) But the longer you stick to a new routine, the easier it will be to resist the old temptations.

> **Make a habit of having fruit for dessert, and it won't take long before you're looking forward to the taste ...**

Become a rebel with a cause

There's another reason that choosing to live healthily is so hard: the world we live in. Some scientists have gone so far as to describe it as a toxic environment because of how it seduces us into making unhealthy choices. Turn on the television, and you'll be besieged

4 INSPIRING TRUTHS ABOUT CHANGE

1 'Human beings, by changing the inner attitudes of their minds, can change the outer aspects of their lives.'
– Psychologist William James

2 'Only I can change my life. No one can do it for me.'
– Actress Carol Burnett

3 'You must be the change you wish to see in the world.'
– Mohandas Gandhi

4 'He that will not apply new remedies, must expect new evils'
– Sir Francis Bacon

with ads for greasy fast foods and sugary cereals. And everywhere you look, new devices are making life more and more sedentary – from people-movers at airports to on-line shopping.

The bottom line is clear: It takes a conscious decision to resist many of the messages being trumpeted around us. The best way to start is to think of yourself as a rebel with a very important cause: your own health and well-being.

Secrets of success

It's not surprising, especially after you discover you have heart trouble, to want to rush in and change everything at once. And, for some people, a crash programme of sweeping reforms works very well. If they have to make adjustments, they say, they'd rather do them all at once.

But there may be a hidden danger in this approach. People who charge ahead in a hurry sometimes have trouble maintaining the changes they've made. To start with, their determination may burn out early, before they've had time to turn their new habits into settled ways of living. What's more, they have a tendency to think of change as all or nothing. And when something comes along that knocks them off track – and almost everyone hits a bump in the road now and then – they can quickly become discouraged, give up and go back to their comfortable old ways.

A surer way to make lasting changes, psychologists say, is step by step, making one moderate change, feeling comfortable with it, and then making another. If you've altered your habits gradually, it may be easier to adjust them when times get hard. If you went from three walks a week to four and then five, it's not a big deal to down-grade to fewer walks when life becomes hectic. And when it eases up, you know what it takes to increase your activities again.

Research in the field of behavioural change has revealed several other strategies that are particularly important to success over the long term. If you take the advice in this book and set out on the path toward a healthier heart, here are five tips to boost your chances of permanent success.

| Make a plan Especially at the beginning, it's easy to feel overwhelmed by all the advice you hear and the changes you want to make. That's why it's important to have a plan for what you want to do – and how you intend to do it. The details should be as

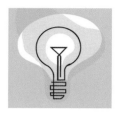

ASK THE EXPERT

**Do some people just have more willpower than others?
Is there anything you can do to increase your willpower?**

Phillip Hodson, Fellow of the British Association of Counselling and Psychotherapy,
and author of many books including *'How perfect is your partner?'*

'It's probably true that some people have more willpower than others. When you're trying to make radical changes to your life, changes that will affect you possibly for the rest of your life, the point is not to depend on willpower – whether you had it in the first place or not.

In everyday language, when we speak of willpower, what we mean is the ability to say no to that tempting chocolate bar, or to walk past the fast-food outlet without going in, no matter how hungry you feel. Or walking the children to school on a rainy day, rather than using the car. The truth is, no matter how much willpower you have, you're bound to falter at some point, and that's more likely to happen if you rely on willpower alone to help you to make a healthy, sensible choice.

Instead, think of willpower as something you fall back on when you really need it. For your everyday life, it's much better to depend on other, more reliable strategies.

Planning is one good example. Decide in advance what you're going to have for lunch, or pack a lunch that's healthy and low in calories. That way you don't have to use your willpower to walk past that fast-food restaurant.

Making sure you have choice is another way to avoid depending on willpower. For instance, if you normally go for a stroll at lunchtime and it's the only time of day that you get any exercise, then a colleague invites you to lunch, you have a crisis of willpower on your hands. You have to decide whether to go for your usual walk or accept an invitation to go out with a friend. But if you also have the option of walking after you get home from work or first thing in the morning, you aren't forced to make a hard decision that requires sheer willpower.

Make sure that you are in a position to be able to call on your willpower whenever it's needed. There are ways to make sure that you can do that.

Getting enough sleep and controlling the stresses in your life are two important ways. It's hard to have enough willpower when you're feeling exhausted or stressed. You'll also strengthen your willpower by remembering why making the healthier choice is important to you.

But don't depend on it and definitely don't use a lack of willpower as an excuse for not being able to adopt new health habits. The real reason people succeed at making lasting changes isn't because they have more willpower than someone else. It's really because they've learnt skills and strategies that allow them to avoid relying solely on their willpower.'

specific as you can make them. 'Eating a healthier diet' just isn't enough. Instead, set a goal of eating at least six servings of fruits and vegetables a day. 'Getting more exercise' isn't specific enough. A better aim would be 'Putting in 40 minutes of walking or climbing on a stair machine five days a week'.

Whatever goals you set, make sure they're realistic. This is not a wish list, it's an action plan. Decide on one or two concrete changes you want to make – then make them. Stick with them until you've successfully introduced the new habits, then tackle others.

Be sure to put your plan in writing, because doing so represents a commitment – a contract with yourself. It should include both long-term goals and interim milestones along the way. One approach is to begin by thinking about where you want to be six months from now. Write down specific goals, such as 'Lose 1½ stones (9kg)' or 'Exercise 5 times a week'. Then break these goals into shorter-term targets for the next month. Finally, work out weekly plans for the coming month that will get you there. See 'A sample plan for heart health', opposite, for an idea of what an effective plan might look like.

2 Chart your progress Once you have your plan drawn up, use a diary or notebook to keep track of your daily progress. The more closely you keep tabs, the better your chances of succeeding. Psychologists call this strategy self-monitoring, and it has proved a remarkably powerful motivational tool. Consider weight loss. Studies show that all people have to do is start keeping a food diary – a detailed accounting of what they eat every day – and they'll begin to lose weight, even if they don't consciously change anything else. This is because keeping a food diary forces you to become more aware of everything you eat during the day. It also helps you spot simple changes you can make to help you to meet your goal.

Finally, charting your progress lets you know when you deserve a pat on the back and spurs you on to greater effort.

3 Find a friend It doesn't matter whether you're trying to stop smoking, eat better, lose weight, exercise more or all of these. If you join forces with someone else who's trying to make the same changes, you'll dramatically improve your chances of success. A study at Indiana University revealed that people

TROUBLESHOOTING TIP

Adopting new habits is tough. One way of making them stick is to practise them daily. Instead of walking for 40 minutes four or five times a week, for instance, aim to walk for 30 minutes every day – rain or shine. Making a daily commitment to yourself leaves less room for procrastination. And the more often you do something, the faster it becomes second nature.

A sample plan for heart health

In a notebook, write down your own heart health game plan using this one as a model. Start with the larger goals you want to accomplish. Next, list actions you're going to take this week. At the end of each week, note your progress. Then formulate your goals for the next week.

MY SIX-MONTH GOALS

1 Lose 1½ stones (9kg)
2 Exercise for 40 minutes a day
3 Eat at least six servings of fruits and vegetables a day

MY ONE-MONTH GOALS

1 Lose 5lb (2.25kg)
2 Walk at least three times a week
3 Look into buying an exercise bike

MY GOALS FOR WEEK 1

1 Take three 15-minute walks this week
2 Have a glass of orange juice or a piece of fruit with cereal every morning
3 Switch from semi-skimmed to skimmed milk

MY GOALS FOR WEEK 2

1 Take three 20-minute walks
2 Try at least one new low-calorie, low-fat recipe for dinner
3 Check out exercise bikes (rent vs. buy)

MY GOALS FOR WEEK 3

1 Take three 25-minute walks
2 Weigh myself to see how I'm doing
3 Make two low-calorie, low-fat recipes for dinner
4 Add a salad or vegetable side dish

MY GOALS FOR WEEK 4

1 Take three 30-minute walks
2 Make low-fat recipes for dinner three times this week
3 Have a serving of fruit every morning for breakfast and at least two vegetables with dinner
4 Make a decision about the exercise bike

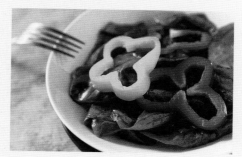

who exercise with a friend are seven times more likely to stick to their plan than those who go it alone. And when researchers at St George's Hospital Medical School at Tooting, in London, paired up smokers trying to kick the habit, they found that the buddy system more than doubled their odds of quitting.

Who should you enlist? Your partner, another family member, a friend, or a colleague may be willing to join you. Many hospitals run support groups for people with heart disease – a great place to find others who want to make the same kind of lifestyle changes. Another option is to talk to your GP. He or she may be able to put you in touch with other heart patients in your area who are looking for company on the path to a healthier life.

If you're looking for moral support, why not explore on-line resources, such as the British Heart Foundation's website at www.bhf.org.uk which includes a great deal of information and advice for both sufferers of heart problems and carers.

4 Look for variety One of the biggest drawbacks people come across over the long term is boredom. If your exercise of choice is walking, you may find yourself getting tired of walking the same route day in and day out. Low-fat meals can be delicious; but if you use the same four or five recipes all the time, dinner is likely to get pretty monotonous.

If you start to feel bored, look for ways to make your new habits interesting again. Find a new place to walk. Better still, take up a new activity. Challenge yourself by joining an exercise class or getting a new bicycle.

Find a way to combine physical activity with something else you love. If you're an avid photographer, for example, take your camera along on walks and be on the lookout for great shots. If you're tired of the same old meals, get a new cookbook that features a cuisine you haven't tried before or sign up for a cooking class. If you have friends who enjoy healthy cooking, what about forming a supper club or a lunch club that allows you to experiment with exciting new dishes together?

5 Keep your eye on your goal The only constant in life is change. As you progress, keep in mind that the things that inspire you to action are likely to change. If you've had a heart attack, you may be motivated first by the fear of having another. As that worry fades, you may find yourself encouraged by the desire to get your old energy back. Now and then, you may not feel very motivated at all. In fact, you may find yourself wondering if

▼ Key finding

Men get more benefit from having an 'exercise buddy' than women do, according to a study done at Ohio State University. Women benefit more from family support. In a poll of 937 randomly selected students, men who exercised regularly reported that they had lots of support from friends who also exercised. Those who rarely worked out reported having few active friends. Physically active women, on the other hand, were much more likely to report being motivated by the encouragement of their families.

all the effort is really worth the trouble. That's why it's so important to keep your eyes on the prize. Remind yourself of why you have you decided to change for the better – to be healthier. But what exactly does that mean?

One measure of health is longevity. We'd all like to enjoy as many healthy years as we can. But since none of us knows how long our lives are meant to be, there's never a moment when we can say, 'Look, I'm enjoying the extra year or two I earned by living a healthier life'.

Of course you'll probably be keeping an eye on other, more objective measures of health – things like weight and cholesterol and blood pressure. They're all important. But over time, they alone aren't usually powerful enough to keep people motivated.

The true reward of living a healthier life, in the end, is how you feel every day. Having the energy to do the things you enjoy without getting tired or experiencing symptoms like shortness of breath or angina; feeling stronger or more capable; and a better mental outlook – being more in control, feeling more confident, enjoying the satisfaction that comes from accomplishing something you set your mind to do.

Some of the rewards you reap may surprise you. You may discover a satisfying hobby that involves a physical activity you never knew you enjoyed. You may learn to enjoy cooking more than you ever thought you could. By enlisting support from friends or colleagues, you may forge new or deeper relationships with others, and by practicing relaxation techniques, you may develop a new sense of inner peace.

In the weeks and months ahead, try to be conscious of all the rewards you are experiencing, large and small. Take time to savour them. Your heart may be the reason you embarked on a healthier lifestyle, but you'll find plenty of other reasons to celebrate your new sense of well-being. And, in turn, by appreciating all the benefits you enjoy, you'll find new sources of motivation and inspiration to keep you on the road to being heart-healthy for life.

> " In the end, the true reward of living a healthier life is how you feel every day. "

RECIPES

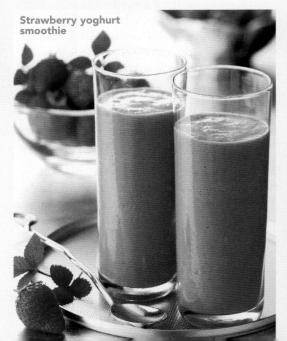

Strawberry yoghurt smoothie

BREAKFAST

Apple and hazelnut drop scones

Drop scones are an almost instant breakfast, made by stirring together a few basic storecupboard ingredients, here with hazelnuts and apples, for extra goodness. Top with a little maple syrup.

Makes 16 scones

45g (1½oz) skinned hazelnuts, chopped
200g (7oz) plain flour
½ tsp bicarbonate of soda
2 tbsp caster sugar
1 large egg
250ml (8½fl oz) buttermilk
1 dessert apple, about 150g (5½oz), cored and finely chopped
1 tbsp sunflower oil
4 tbsp maple syrup

Preparation time: 15 minutes

1 Heat a small non-stick frying pan, add the hazelnuts and cook until golden brown, stirring and tossing constantly. Take care not to overcook the nuts as they burn easily. Tip them into a small bowl.

2 Sift the flour, bicarbonate of soda, salt and sugar into a large mixing bowl. Make a well in the centre. Lightly beat the egg with the buttermilk and pour into the well. Gradually whisk the flour mixture into the buttermilk mixture to make a smooth, thick batter. Add the apple and toasted hazelnuts, and stir in with a large metal spoon.

3 Lightly brush a griddle or heavy frying pan with a little of the sunflower oil, then heat over a moderate heat. Depending on the size of the griddle or pan, you can cook about 4 scones at the same time. For each one, drop 1 heaped tbsp of batter onto the hot surface. Bubbles will rise to the surface and burst. Gently slip a small palette knife under the drop scone to loosen it, then cook for a further minute or until the underside is golden brown. Turn the scone over and cook the other side for 1–2 minutes or until golden.

4 Remove the scones from the griddle or frying pan and keep warm under a clean cloth. Cook the rest of the batter in the same way.

5 When all the drop scones are cooked, quickly heat the maple syrup in a small saucepan just to warm it. Drizzle the syrup over the warm drop scones and serve immediately.

EACH SERVING PROVIDES:
kcal 106, **protein** 3g, **fat** 3g (of which saturated fat 0.5g), **carbohydrate** 18g (of which sugars 8g), **fibre** 1g

Strawberry yoghurt smoothie

This refreshing drink – full of vitamin C – takes only a few minutes to prepare. So it's ideal to start the day or as a light snack at any time.

Serves 4

450g (1lb) ripe strawberries, hulled
grated zest and juice of 1 large orange
150g (5½oz) plain low-fat yoghurt
1 tbsp caster sugar, or to taste (optional)
TO DECORATE (optional)
4 small strawberries
4 small slices of orange

Preparation time: 5 minutes

1 Tip the strawberries into a food processor or blender and add the grated orange zest, orange juice and yoghurt. Blend to a smooth purée, scraping down the sides of the container once or twice. Taste the mixture and sweeten with the sugar, if necessary.

2 For a really smooth consistency, press through a nylon sieve to remove the strawberry pips, although this is not essential.

3 Pour into glasses. If you like, decorate with small strawberries and slices of orange, both split so they sit on the rim of the glass.

EACH SERVING PROVIDES:
kcal 55, **protein** 3g, **fat** 0.5g (of which saturated fat 0.2g), **carbohydrate** 11g (of which sugars 11g), **fibre** 1g

Fruity Bircher muesli

A delicious toasted muesli, this is made from a mix of grains, nuts, seeds and colourful berries. Stirring maple syrup and orange juice into the mix helps to keep the oil content down.

Makes 500g (1lb 2oz)

225g (8oz) rolled oats
45g (1½oz) wheatgerm
55g (2oz) millet flakes
1 tbsp sesame seeds
2 tbsp sunflower seeds
2 tbsp slivered almonds
50g (1¾oz) dried blueberries
50g (1¾oz) dried cranberries
15g (½oz) soft brown or demerara sugar
2 tbsp maple syrup
2 tbsp sunflower oil
2 tbsp orange juice

Preparation time: 10 minutes, plus overnight soaking

1 Preheat the oven to 160°C (325°F, gas mark 3). In a large bowl, combine the oats, wheatgerm, millet flakes, sesame and sunflower seeds, almonds, dried berries and sugar. Stir until well mixed.

2 Put the maple syrup, oil and orange juice in a small jug and whisk together. Pour this mixture slowly into the dry ingredients, stirring to ensure that the liquid is evenly distributed and coats everything lightly.

3 Spread the mixture out evenly in a non-stick roasting tin. Bake for 30–40 minutes or until slightly crisp and lightly browned. Stir the mixture every 10 minutes to encourage even browning.

4 Remove from the oven and leave to cool. Store in an airtight container for up to 2 weeks. Serve with yoghurt, milk or fruit juice.

EACH SERVING PROVIDES:
kcal 250, **protein** 7g, **fat** 11g (of which saturated fat 0.8g), **carbohydrate** 32g (of which sugars 7g), **fibre** 4g

SALADS

Bulghur wheat and prawn salad

A coarsely ground wheat grain, bulghur has already been parboiled, so it's quick to prepare and makes a healthy storecupboard standby.

Serves 4

250g (8½oz) bulghur wheat
1 small red onion, very thinly sliced
1 carrot, coarsely grated
1 tomato, diced
6 baby corn, sliced into rounds
½ cucumber, diced
200g (7oz) peeled cooked prawns
LIME AND CHILLI DRESSING
4 tbsp extra virgin olive oil
2 tbsp lime juice
1 garlic clove, crushed
¼ tsp crushed dried chillies

Preparation and cooking time: 20–25 minutes

1 Put the bulghur wheat in a saucepan and pour over 650ml (22fl oz) water. Bring to the boil, then simmer for 10 minutes or until the bulghur is tender and all the water has been absorbed. Tip the bulghur into a flat dish, spread out and allow to cool slightly.

2 Combine the onion, carrot, tomato, corn, cucumber and prawns in a large salad bowl. Add the bulghur wheat and stir together.

3 For the dressing, put the oil, lime juice, garlic, crushed chilli, and salt and pepper to taste in a small bowl. Whisk with a fork until combined. Stir the dressing into the salad, tossing to coat all the ingredients evenly. If you are not serving the salad immediately, cover and keep in the fridge.

EACH SERVING PROVIDES:
kcal 399, **protein** 19g, **fat** 13g (of which saturated fat 2g), **carbohydrate** 53g (of which sugars 5g), **fibre** 2g

Avocado salad with raspberries

Avocados contain quite a lot of fat but it is the heart-friendly monounsaturated type. Here, the creaminess of avocado is complemented by fresh raspberries and a fruity vinaigrette.

Serves 4

2 avocados
170g (6oz) mixed salad leaves, such as
        frisée, baby chard and lamb's lettuce
100g (3½oz) raspberries
sprigs of fresh mint to garnish

RASPBERRY VINAIGRETTE
2 tbsp extra virgin olive oil
1½ tbsp raspberry vinegar
1 tbsp single cream
finely grated zest of ½ orange
½ tsp orange juice
pinch of caster sugar

Preparation time: about 10 minutes

1 Put all the ingredients for the vinaigrette in a large salad bowl, adding salt and pepper to taste, and whisk to mix.

2 Halve the avocados and remove the stone, then peel and dice the flesh. Drop immediately into the dressing and turn to coat, to prevent the avocado from turning brown.

3 Add the salad leaves to the bowl and toss gently with the avocado. Scatter over the raspberries and garnish with mint sprigs. Serve at once.

EACH SERVING PROVIDES:
kcal 255, **protein** 3g, **fat** 25g (of which saturated fat 5g), **carbohydrate** 4g (of which sugars 3g), **fibre** 4g

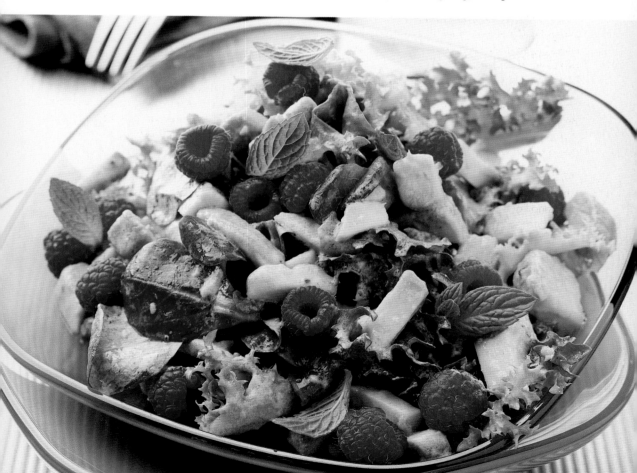

Sprouted bean salad

The nutritional content of pulses and grains increases dramatically when they are sprouted – there is 60 per cent more vitamin C and almost 30 per cent more B vitamins in the sprout than the original seed. Choose fresh-looking, crisp sprouts, preferably with the seed still attached. They will keep for up to 2 days in a plastic bag in the fridge.

Serves 4

55g (2oz) dried apricots, chopped
125g (4½oz) dried mango, chopped
4 tbsp apple juice
2 courgettes, cut into 1cm (½in) dice
2 small heads chicory, halved lengthways and
    sliced across
300g (10½oz) assorted bean and grain
    sprouts, such as mung, aduki and alfalfa
DRESSING
30g (1oz) fresh root ginger, peeled
    and finely chopped
1 tsp wholegrain mustard
2 tsp cider vinegar
2 tsp clear honey
3 tbsp sunflower oil
1 tbsp poppy seeds

Preparation time:
25 minutes, plus 1 hour soaking

1 Put the dried apricots and mango in a salad bowl and spoon over the apple juice. Cover and leave to soak for 1 hour or until the juice has been soaked up and the fruit is plump.

2 Add the courgettes, chicory, and bean and grain sprouts, and toss together to mix thoroughly.

3 To make the dressing, first press the ginger in a garlic press until you have 2 tsp of ginger juice. Then whisk this juice with the mustard, vinegar, honey and salt and pepper to taste. Gradually add the oil, whisking until slightly thickened. Stir in the poppy seeds. Pour the dressing over the salad, toss and serve at once.

EACH SERVING PROVIDES:
kcal 290, protein 11g, fat 14g (of which saturated fat 6g), carbohydrate 34g (of which sugars 2g), fibre 2g

---

SANDWICHES

Ham and celeriac pittas

This refreshing salad sandwich is packed with a mixture of crunchy vegetables, smoked ham, dried fruit and green olives that gives lovely contrasting flavours and textures. The tangy mustard dressing is based on Greek-style yoghurt and mayonnaise. Add a piece of fresh fruit and you have a really healthy lunch.

Serves 6

125g (4½oz) piece celeriac
2 carrots, about 150g (5½oz) in total
170g (6oz) thickly sliced lean smoked ham,
    cut into 1cm (½in) dice
1 small red onion, thinly sliced
8 stoned green olives, pimento-stuffed
    if desired, halved
50g (1¾oz) currants
2 tbsp chopped parsley
6 garlic pitta breads
1 heart of romaine or cos lettuce, finely shredded
parsley to garnish
MUSTARD DRESSING
3 tbsp Greek-style yoghurt
½ tsp wholegrain mustard
2 tbsp mayonnaise

Preparation time: 15 minutes

1 Preheat the grill to high. Mix together all the dressing ingredients in a medium-sized bowl.

2 Peel and coarsely grate the celeriac and carrots. Add to the bowl of dressing and mix well. Add the ham, onion, olives, currants and chopped parsley and mix everything together.

3 Warm the pitta breads under the grill for about 1 minute on each side. Cut each one across in half to make 2 pockets of bread. Divide the lettuce among the pitta pockets, then add the ham and celeriac salad. Garnish with parsley and serve.

EACH SERVING PROVIDES:
kcal 320, protein 13g, fat 6g (of which saturated fat 1g), carbohydrate 54g (of which sugars 11g), fibre 3g

Hot and spicy tuna rolls

Here, the soft interiors of large crusty bread rolls are hollowed out to provide a crisp casing for a gently spiced mix of tuna, sweetcorn and red kidney beans, and then warmed in the oven. For a light lunch that is satisfying and well-balanced, serve with a mixed tomato and leaf salad.

Serves 4

4 large, rounded, crusty white bread rolls, about 10cm (4in) across, about 100g (3½oz) each
2 tbsp soured cream
2 tbsp mayonnaise
1 tsp hot or medium chilli sauce
2 tsp lime juice
1 can tuna in spring water, about 200g, drained
1 can sweetcorn, about 200g, drained
1 can red kidney beans, about 200g, drained and rinsed
½ green pepper, seeded and diced
2 tbsp chopped fresh coriander

Preparation time: 15 minutes
Cooking time: 10 minutes

1 Preheat the oven to 180°C (350°F, gas mark 4). Slice the tops off the bread rolls and set aside. Scoop out most of the soft interior, leaving a 'shell' about 1cm (½in) thick. Place the hollowed-out rolls on one side with the bread lids.

2 Make the scooped-out bread into crumbs, either by crumbling with your fingers or using a food processor. Spread 85g (3oz) of the breadcrumbs on a baking tray and toast in the oven for 10 minutes or until dry and crisp. Remove from the oven and set aside. Leave the oven on.

3 Mix together the soured cream, mayonnaise, chilli sauce and lime juice. Add the tuna, sweet-corn, red kidney beans, green pepper, coriander and dried breadcrumbs. Season with salt and pepper to taste. Mix together, taking care not to break up the chunks of tuna too much.

4 Spoon the tuna mixture into the hollowed-out rolls and replace the lids. Set on the baking tray and cover loosely with foil. Bake for 5 minutes, then remove the foil and bake for a further 5 minutes, to crisp the bread crust. The filling should be warm, but not bubbling. Serve immediately.

EACH SERVING PROVIDES
kcal 449, **protein** 22g, **fat** 12.5g (of which saturated fat 4 g), **carbohydrate** 67g (of which sugars 8g), **fibre** 9g

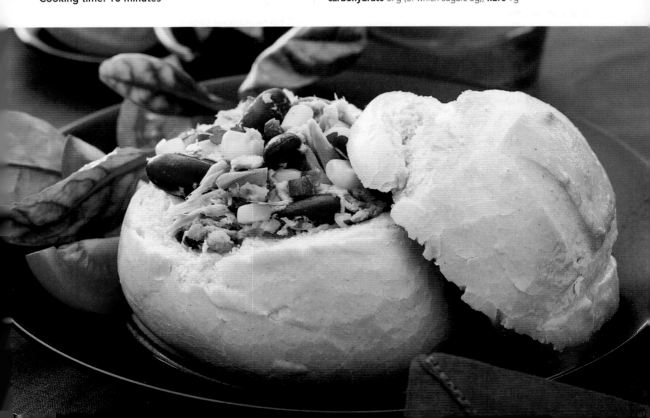

Golden lentil soup

This velvety-smooth soup owes its rich colour to a combination of lentils, parsnips and carrots. With dry sherry and a horseradish-flavoured cream adding to the flavour, it is a perfect dinner-party first course. Serve it with crunchy melba toast or oatcakes.

Serves 6

30g (1oz) butter
1 large onion, finely chopped
450g (1lb) parsnips, cut into small cubes
340g (12oz) carrots, cut into small cubes
150ml (5fl oz) dry sherry

85g (3oz) red lentils
1.2 litres (2 pints) vegetable stock
fresh chives to garnish
TO SERVE
2 tsp grated horseradish
6 tbsp crème fraîche

Preparation time: about 15 minutes
Cooking time: about 1¼ hours

1 Melt the butter in a large saucepan. Add the onion, stir well and cover the pan. Sweat the onion over a gentle heat for 10 minutes or until softened. Stir in the parsnips, carrots and sherry. Bring to the boil, then cover the pan again and leave to simmer very gently for 40 minutes.

2 Add the lentils, stock, and salt and pepper to taste. Bring to the boil, then reduce the heat and cover the pan. Simmer for a further 15–20 minutes or until the lentils are tender. Purée the soup in a blender until smooth or use a hand-held blender to purée the soup in the pan. Return the soup to the pan if necessary, and reheat it gently until boiling. If it seems a bit thick, add a little stock or water.

3 Stir the grated horseradish into the crème fraîche. Snip some of the chives for the garnish and leave a few whole. Ladle the soup into warm bowls and top each portion with a spoonful of the horseradish cream. Scatter snipped chives over the top and add a few lengths of whole chive across the top of each bowl. Serve at once.

EACH SERVING PROVIDES:
kcal 250, protein 6g, **fat** 11g (of which saturated fat 3g), **carbohydrate** 25g (of which sugars 11g), **fibre** 6g

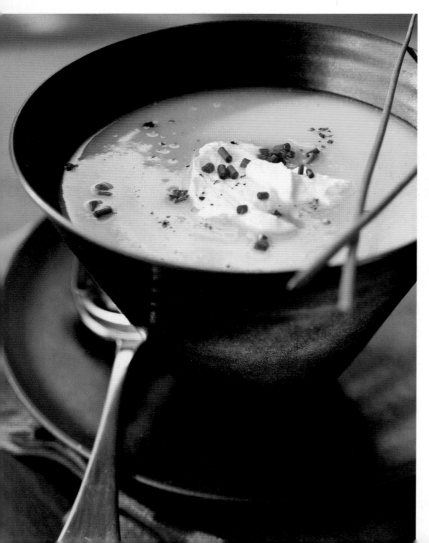

Japanese miso soup

Ginger, shiitake mushrooms and a stock made with dried kombu seaweed bring rich savoury flavours to this Oriental broth, which is quick, easy to make and ideal for a healthy first course.

Serves 4

1 packet dried kombu seaweed, about 25g
1 tbsp sake, Chinese rice wine or dry sherry
2 tsp caster sugar
½ tsp finely grated fresh root ginger
2 tbsp miso paste
4 spring onions, sliced at an angle
6 fresh shiitake mushrooms, thinly sliced
85g (3oz) tofu, diced
85g (3oz) watercress leaves

Preparation time: 10 minutes, plus 5 minutes soaking
Cooking time: about 20 minutes

1 Put the kombu seaweed in a saucepan and pour in 1 litre (1¾ pints) water. Bring slowly to the boil, then remove from the heat and cover the pan. Set aside for 5 minutes. Use a draining spoon to remove and discard the kombu seaweed.

2 Stir the sake, rice wine or sherry, sugar and ginger into the broth and bring back to the boil. Reduce the heat, and stir in the miso paste until it dissolves completely.

3 Add the spring onions, mushrooms, tofu and watercress. Cook very gently, stirring, for 2 minutes without allowing the soup to boil. Ladle the soup into small bowls and serve at once.

EACH SERVING PROVIDES:
kcal 55, **protein** 3g, **fat** 2g (of which saturated fat 0g), **carbohydrate** 5.5g (of which sugars 5g), **fibre** 4g

Classic gazpacho

This traditional Spanish soup is full of fresh flavours and packed with vitamins as all the vegetables are raw. It is ideal for a simple lunch or supper, served with some crusty country-style bread or rolls and would also make an excellent light starter.

Serves 4

500g (1lb 2oz) full-flavoured tomatoes,
    quartered and seeded
¼ cucumber, peeled and coarsely chopped
1 medium-sized red pepper, seeded and
    coarsely chopped
2 garlic cloves
1 small onion, quartered
1 slice of bread, about 30g (1oz),
    torn into pieces
2 tbsp red wine vinegar
2 tbsp extra virgin olive oil
500ml (17fl oz) tomato juice
1 tbsp tomato purée
TO SERVE
1 red pepper
4 spring onions
¼ cucumber
2 slices of bread, made into croutons

Preparation time: 20 minutes,
    plus 2 hours chilling

1 Mix all the ingredients in a large bowl. Ladle batches of the mixture into a blender and purée until smooth. Pour the soup into a large clean bowl, cover and chill for 2 hours.

2 Prepare the vegetables to serve with the soup towards the end of the chilling time. Seed and finely dice the red pepper; thinly slice the spring onions; and finely dice the cucumber. Place these vegetables and the croutons in separate serving dishes.

3 Taste the soup and adjust the seasoning, then ladle it into bowls. Serve at once, offering the accompaniments so that they can be added to taste as the soup is eaten.

EACH SERVING PROVIDES:
kcal 215, **protein** 6g, **fat** 9g (of which saturated fat 1.5g), **carbohydrate** 30g (of which sugars 17g), **fibre** 5g

DINNER

Pork steaks with mustard sauce

This delectable dish is surprisingly easy to make. Serve with boiled potatoes sprinkled with chives, steamed carrots and shredded Savoy cabbage.

Serves 4

1 tsp extra virgin olive oil
4 boneless pork loin steaks or chops,
    1.5–2cm (⅝–¾in) thick, about 550g
    (1¼lb) in total, trimmed of all fat
4 tbsp dry white wine or vermouth
1 garlic clove, finely chopped
170ml (6fl oz) chicken or vegetable stock
2 tsp cornflour mixed with 1 tbsp water
120ml (4fl oz) crème fraîche
1 tbsp Dijon mustard
1 tbsp chopped fresh tarragon
fresh chives to garnish

Preparation and cooking time: 30 minutes

1 Heat the oil in a non-stick frying pan over a moderately high heat. Add the pork steaks and fry for 3 minutes on each side or until well browned. Put the steaks on a plate, and keep on one side.

2 Add the wine or vermouth to the frying pan with the garlic and let it bubble briefly, then pour in the stock and boil for 2 minutes. Stir together the cornflour mixture and crème fraîche until smooth. Add to the hot cooking liquid, stirring well. Simmer gently for 2 minutes, stirring constantly, until it is thickened and smooth. Then stir in the mustard and tarragon, and season with salt and pepper to taste.

3 Return the pork steaks to the sauce. Reduce the heat to low, cover the pan and cook for 4–5 minutes or until the steaks are cooked through.

4 Arrange the pork steaks on warm plates and spoon the sauce over. Garnish and serve at once.

EACH SERVING PROVIDES:
kcal 325, **protein** 31g, **fat** 20g (of which saturated fat 7g), **carbohydrate** 4g (of which sugars 1g), **fibre** 0g

Thai-style stir-fried beef with mango

This colourful Oriental dish is bursting with fresh flavours and contrasting textures. Although a little oil is used to stir-fry the beef, the dressing is oil-free so the dish is still very light in fat.

Serves 4

400g (14oz) lean steak,
    such as sirloin
3 garlic cloves, finely chopped
1 tsp caster sugar
2 tsp soy sauce
1½ tbsp sunflower oil
GINGER AND HONEY DRESSING
2 tsp paprika
2 tsp mild Mexican-style chilli powder
1½ tbsp clear honey
2.5cm (1in) piece fresh root ginger, grated
4 tbsp rice vinegar or cider vinegar
juice of 1 lime or lemon

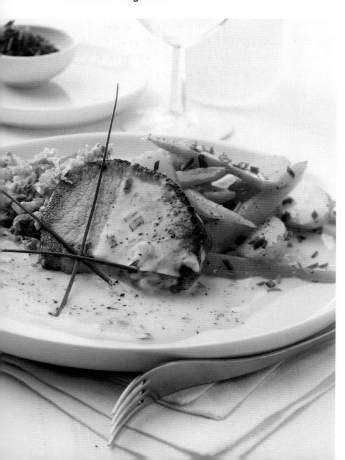

SALAD

1 ripe but firm mango, peeled and cut into strips
2 ripe but firm plums, sliced
¼ medium-sized red cabbage, shredded
55g (2oz) watercress leaves
½ cucumber, cut into matchsticks
½ red pepper, cut into thin strips
3–4 spring onions, cut into diagonal pieces
45g (1½oz) mixed fresh mint and coriander
2 tbsp coarsely chopped roasted unsalted peanuts

Preparation time: 30 minutes
Cooking time: about 10 minutes

1 To make the dressing, put the paprika, chilli powder, honey, ginger and vinegar in a saucepan and slowly add 250ml (8½fl oz) of water, stirring. Bring to the boil, then reduce the heat and simmer for 5 minutes. Remove from the heat and stir in the lime or lemon juice. Set aside.

2 Combine all the salad ingredients, except the peanuts, in a large shallow serving dish and toss gently together until evenly mixed. Set aside.

3 Cut the steak into thin strips for stir-frying. Put the steak in a bowl with the garlic, sugar and soy sauce and mix together so that the strips of steak are seasoned. Heat a wok or non-stick pan on a high heat, then add the oil. Add the beef and stir-fry until the strips are evenly browned and cooked to taste.

4 Spoon the stir-fried beef over the top of the salad. Drizzle the dressing over the top and sprinkle with the peanuts. Serve immediately.

EACH SERVING PROVIDES:
kcal 265, **protein** 27g, **fat** 8g (of which saturated fat 3g), **carbohydrate** 20g (of which sugars 18g), **fibre** 3g

Pan-fried turkey escalopes with citrus honey sauce

The tanginess of citrus fruit marries extremely well with poultry. Here, orange, lemon, honey and shallots, create a tasty sauce for turkey escalopes, served on a stack of green beans. For a simple accompaniment, steam some new potatoes.

Serves 4

4 small skinless turkey breast steaks, about 115g (4oz) each
30g (1oz) butter
4 large shallots, thinly sliced
1 garlic clove, crushed
400g (14oz) fine French beans, trimmed
2 tbsp clear honey
grated zest and juice of 1 orange
grated zest and juice of 1 lemon

Preparation time: 15 minutes
Cooking time: about 15 minutes

1 Put the turkey steaks between sheets of cling film and pound them to flatten to about 5mm (¼in) thickness. Set these escalopes aside.

2 Melt the butter in a large frying pan, add the shallots and garlic, and cook, stirring, for 2–3 minutes or until softened but not brown. Remove the shallots from the pan with a draining spoon and set aside.

3 Put the turkey escalopes in the pan, in one layer, and fry them for 2–3 minutes on each side.

4 Meanwhile, cook the beans in a saucepan of boiling salted water for 3–4 minutes or until just tender. Drain and rinse briefly in cold water to stop the cooking. Keep the beans warm.

5 Mix the honey with the zest and juice of the orange and lemon. Remove the turkey escalopes from the pan and keep hot. Pour the honey mixture into the pan, return the shallots and garlic, and add seasoning to taste. Bring to the boil and bubble for about 2 minutes, stirring constantly.

6 Make a pile of beans on 4 plates and place a turkey escalope on top of each pile. Spoon over the sliced shallots and pan juices, and serve.

EACH SERVING PROVIDES:
kcal 245, **protein** 27g, **fat** 9g (of which saturated fat 5g), **carbohydrate** 14g (of which sugars 13g), **fibre** 2.5g

Basil-stuffed chicken breasts

This stylish main course is, surprisingly, not laden with fat. The chicken breasts can be prepared in advance and kept, covered, in the fridge. You could serve it with tagliatelle tossed with a little grated lemon zest, plus a bread such as ciabatta.

Serves 4

4 skinless boneless chicken breasts (fillets), about 140g (5oz) each
100g (3½oz) mozzarella cheese, thinly sliced
1 tomato, thinly sliced
1 garlic clove, crushed
1 bunch of fresh basil, about 20g (¾oz)
4 slices Parma ham, about 55g (2oz) in total
1 tbsp extra virgin olive oil
GREEN SALAD
2 tbsp extra virgin olive oil
juice of ½ lemon
125g (4½oz) pack gourmet lettuce selection or mixed salad leaves
1 bunch of watercress, large stalks discarded

Preparation time: 25–30 minutes
Cooking time: about 15 minutes

1 Preheat the oven to 220°C (425°F, gas mark 7). Make a slit along the length of each chicken breast and enlarge to form a pocket.

2 Divide the mozzarella among the chicken breasts, sliding the slices into the pockets. Top the cheese with the tomato slices and crushed garlic. Roughly chop a little of the basil and add to each pocket.

3 Season each chicken breast. Place a large sprig of basil on each, then wrap in a slice of Parma ham, making sure the ham covers the slit in the chicken. Tie the ham securely in place with three or four pieces of string on each breast.

4 Heat the oil in a heavy-based frying pan (preferably one with an ovenproof handle). Add the chicken breasts and fry over a high heat for 3–4 minutes, turning to brown both sides.

5 Transfer the pan to the oven (or transfer the chicken to an oven dish) and bake for 10–12 minutes or until the chicken is cooked through; the juices should run clear when the thickest part of the chicken is pierced with a knife.

6 Meanwhile, make the salad. Put the oil and lemon juice in a bowl, season and mix well together. Add the lettuce and watercress. Toss, then divide among 4 serving plates.

7 Remove the string from the chicken breasts. Cut each breast across into slices, holding it together so it keeps its shape. Place on the salad and garnish with the remaining basil.

EACH SERVING PROVIDES:
kcal 339, **protein** 40g, **fat** 19g (of which saturated fat 6g), **carbohydrate** 1.5g (of which sugars 1g), **fibre** 1g

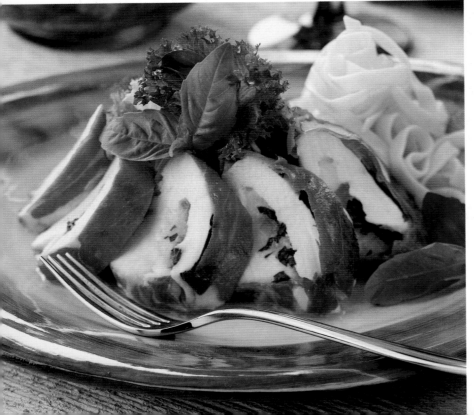

Summer salmon and asparagus

Fresh young vegetables and succulent salmon make this casserole highly nutritious and it is also quick to prepare. Choose tiny leeks, tender asparagus, sugarsnap peas, which all look superb, and boiled new potatoes to complete the meal.

Serves 4

4 pieces skinless salmon fillets,
     about 140g (5oz) each
200g (7oz) baby leeks
250g (8½oz) tender asparagus spears
150g (5½oz) sugarsnap peas
4 tbsp dry white wine
200ml (7fl oz) fish or vegetable stock
30g (1oz) butter, cut into small pieces
1 tbsp snipped fresh chives to garnish

Preparation time: 10 minutes
Cooking time: about 20 minutes

1 Run your fingertips over each salmon fillet to check for stray bones, pulling out any that remain between the flakes of fish. Arrange the leeks in a single layer in the bottom of a large, shallow flame-proof casserole. Lay the pieces of salmon on top. Surround the fish with the asparagus and sugar-snap peas. Pour in the wine and stock, and dot the butter over the fish. Season with salt and pepper.

2 Bring to a boil, then cover the casserole with a tight-fitting lid and reduce the heat so the liquid simmers gently. Cook the fish and vegetables for 12-14 minutes or until the salmon is pale pink all the way through and the vegetables are tender. Sprinkle the chives over the salmon and serve.

EACH SERVING PROVIDES:
kcal 360, **protein** 33g, **fat** 22g (of which saturated fat 7g), **carbohydrate** 4g (of which sugars 4g), **fibre** 3g

Tagliatelle with green sauce

This simple vegetable and yoghurt sauce is bursting with fresh flavours and irresistibly creamy, though it is much lighter than the classic cream sauce for pasta. A salad of crisp radicchio and Lollo Rosso lettuce completes the meal.

Serves 4

225g (8oz) baby spinach, thick stalks discarded
100g (3½oz) watercress, thick stalks discarded
125g (4½oz) frozen peas
500g (1lb 2oz) fresh tagliatelle
2 tsp cornflour
200ml (7fl oz) Greek-style yoghurt
4 tbsp chopped parsley
6 sprigs of fresh basil, torn into pieces

Preparation time: 5 minutes
Cooking time: 7–8 minutes

1 Rinse the spinach and watercress and place in a large saucepan with just the water clinging to the leaves. Cover and cook over a moderate heat for 2 minutes, stirring and turning the vegetables occasionally, until they have wilted.

2 Add the peas and heat through, uncovered, for 2 minutes – there should be enough liquid in the pan to cook the peas. Tip the greens and their liquid into a bowl. Set aside.

3 Cook the pasta in a large saucepan of boiling water for 3 minutes, or according to the packet instructions, until al dente.

4 Meanwhile, blend the cornflour to a smooth paste with the yoghurt, and put into the pan used for cooking the vegetables. Stir over a moderate heat until just bubbling. Add the vegetables, parsley, basil and seasoning to taste and stir well. Heat the sauce through, then remove the pan from the heat.

5 Drain the pasta and add to the sauce. Toss to mix with the sauce, then serve.

(V) EACH SERVING PROVIDES:
kcal 215, **protein** 11g, **fat** 6g (of which saturated fat 3g), **carbohydrate** 30g (of which sugars 3g), **fibre** 4g

Sun-dried tomato and bean risotto

Moist risotto served with a simple side salad makes a satisfying carbohydrate-rich meal, and the risotto can be endlessly varied – all sorts of other vegetables (fresh, frozen, canned or dried) can be used instead of broad beans. To achieve the perfect texture, use risotto rice such as arborio and add the hot stock in stages.

Serves 4

1 tbsp extra virgin olive oil
1 large onion, chopped
2 garlic cloves, crushed
300g (10½oz) risotto rice
85g (3oz) sun-dried tomatoes (dry-packed),
       coarsely chopped
240ml (8fl oz) dry white wine
1.2 litres (2 pints) hot vegetable stock,
       preferably homemade
225g (8oz) frozen broad beans
55g (2oz) Parmesan cheese, freshly grated
30g (1oz) pine nuts
TO GARNISH
12 large fresh basil leaves, shredded,

Preparation time: 5 minutes
Cooking time: 25 minutes

1 Heat the oil in a large saucepan. Add the onion and garlic and fry over a moderate heat for 5 minutes, stirring frequently, until the onion softens and begins to colour.

2 Stir in the rice and sun-dried tomatoes, making sure the grains are coated in the oil, then pour in the wine. Bring to the boil, stirring occasionally.

3 Pour in half the hot stock and bring back to the boil, then reduce the heat and simmer, stirring frequently, for 10 minutes. Add the broad beans and half the remaining hot stock. Bring back to the boil again, then continue to simmer for about 10 minutes, adding the remaining stock in one or two stages as the rice absorbs the liquid.

4 The risotto is ready when the rice is tender but the grains are still whole, and the broad beans are cooked. It should be moist and creamy.

5 Add the Parmesan cheese and pine nuts with seasoning to taste and stir to mix. Serve at once, sprinkled with shredded basil.

(V) **EACH SERVING PROVIDES:**
kcal 610, **protein** 17g, **fat** 25g (of which saturated fat 5g), **carbohydrate** 67g (of which sugars 5g), **fibre** 4g

Noodles with roasted vegetables

Oven-roasted vegetables, tender and scented with garlic, make a chunky dressing that is great with wide pasta noodles. A sprinkling of crunchy sunflower seeds adds texture as well as additional nutritional benefits.

Serves 4

1 aubergine, cut into large chunks
2 courgettes, cut into large chunks
2 red peppers, quartered and seeded
1 green pepper, quartered and seeded
4 ripe tomatoes, halved
2 red onions, quartered
1 head garlic, cloves separated but unpeeled,
       plus 2 garlic cloves, chopped
3 tbsp extra virgin olive oil
cayenne pepper
50g (1¾oz) sunflower seeds
soy sauce
340g (12oz) wide pasta noodles, such as
       reginette, lasagnette or pappardelle
3 tbsp tomato purée, or to taste
handful of fresh basil leaves, coarsely chopped
       if large, or 2 tbsp chopped fresh parsley

Preparation time: about 20 minutes
Cooking time: about 45 minutes

1 Preheat the oven to 190°C (375°F, gas mark 5). Arrange the aubergine, courgettes, red and green peppers, tomatoes, red onions and whole garlic cloves in a single layer in a large ovenproof dish or roasting tin. Sprinkle with about 2 tbsp of the olive oil, a little cayenne pepper, half the chopped garlic, and salt and pepper.

2 Roast for about 45 minutes or until all the vegetables are tender but not soft and mushy, and are charred in places. Turn the vegetables once or twice during cooking, and increase the heat slightly if they are not cooking quickly enough.

3 Meanwhile, toast the sunflower seeds. Lightly brush a frying pan with just a few drops of olive oil, then heat the pan. Add the sunflower seeds and toss and turn them for a few moments until they begin to toast. Shake in a few drops of soy sauce and turn the seeds quickly, letting the soy sauce evaporate as the seeds toast and brown lightly. This should take about 4–5 minutes in total. Remove from the heat just before the seeds are crisp and leave them to cool in the pan. They will crisp up as they cool.

4 Cook the pasta in boiling water for 10–12 minutes, or according to the packet instructions, until al dente. Drain well and keep hot.

5 Using a knife and fork, cut the roasted vegetables into bite-sized chunks. Toss the vegetables and garlic with the remaining raw chopped garlic, the tomato purée and basil or parsley. Taste for seasoning.

6 Toss the pasta with the vegetables and serve at once, sprinkled with the toasted sunflower seeds.

(v) **EACH SERVING PROVIDES:**
kcal 530, **protein** 17g, **fat** 17g (of which saturated fat 2g), **carbohydrate** 83g (of which sugars 16g), **fibre** 8.5g

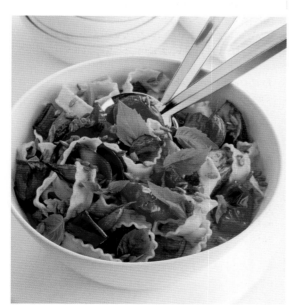

VEGETABLES

Roast root vegetables with herbs

Use this recipe as a basic guide for roasting single vegetables, such as potatoes or parsnips, as well as for a superb dish of mixed roots. Serve them in generous quantities with a main dish.

Serves 4

1kg (2¼lb) root vegetables, such as potatoes, carrots, parsnips and swede
225g (8oz) shallots or pickling onions
2 tbsp extra virgin olive oil
1 tsp cracked black peppercorns
few sprigs of fresh thyme
few sprigs of fresh rosemary

Preparation time: 15–20 minutes
Cooking time: 30–35 minutes

1 Preheat the oven to 220°C (425°F, gas mark 7). Scrub or peel the vegetables, according to type and your taste. Halve or quarter large potatoes. Cut large carrots or parsnips in half lengthways, then cut the pieces across in half again. Cut swede or kohlrabi into large chunks (about the same size as the potatoes). Leave shallots or onions whole.

2 Place the vegetables in a saucepan and pour in enough boiling water to cover them. Bring back to the boil, then reduce the heat and simmer for 5–7 minutes or until the vegetables are lightly cooked, but not yet tender.

3 Drain the vegetables and place in a roasting tin. Brush with the oil and sprinkle with salt (if desired) and peppercorns. Add the herb sprigs to the tin and place in the oven.

4 Roast for 30–35 minutes or until the vegetables are golden brown, crisp and tender. Turn them over halfway through the cooking. Serve hot, garnished with sprigs of thyme or rosemary, if liked.

EACH SERVING PROVIDES:
kcal 200, **protein** 4g, **fat** 7g (of which saturated fat 1g), **carbohydrate** 33g (of which sugars 14g), **fibre** 7g

Baked pumpkin with red onion and sage

Pumpkin is an easy-to-cook accompaniment for all sorts of main dishes, as are the other squashes that can be used in this recipe. Club-shaped butternut squash is available for most of the year, and in autumn there are small acorn squash, kabocha squash and the Prince Regent squash with its eggshell blue skin.

Serves 4

1 small pumpkin, about 1.6kg (3½lb), peeled, seeded and cubed, or 900g (2lb) prepared pumpkin flesh, cubed
2 red onions, cut into wedges
4 garlic cloves, thinly sliced
3 tbsp chopped fresh sage
2 tbsp extra virgin olive oil

Preparation time: 20–25 minutes
Cooking time: 35 minutes

1 Preheat the oven to 220°C (425°F, gas mark 7). Lay a large sheet of foil on a baking tray. Pile the pumpkin and onions in the middle of the foil. Alternatively, prepare 4 sheets of foil and cook the pumpkin in individual parcels.

2 Scatter the garlic and sage over the pumpkin, then drizzle the oil over and add seasoning to taste. Fold up the foil to enclose the pumpkin, then fold the edges together to seal the vegetables inside a neat parcel.

3 Bake the pumpkin parcel or parcels for 30 minutes, then open the foil and bake for a further 5 minutes or until the pumpkin is tender and beginning to brown. Serve hot.

(V) **EACH SERVING PROVIDES:**
kcal 115, **protein** 3g, **fat** 6g (of which saturated fat 1g), **carbohydrate** 12g (of which sugars 8g), **fibre** 5g

Sesame greens and bean sprouts

With a little inspiration and the availability of international ingredients, even the most humble vegetables can be elevated to feature in unusual, well-flavoured side dishes. This succulent stir-fry is full of flavour and crunch. It is ideal as part of an Oriental menu or equally delicious with plain grilled fish, poultry or meat.

Serves 4

30g (1oz) sesame seeds
2 tbsp sunflower oil
1 onion, chopped
2 garlic cloves, chopped
1 small Savoy cabbage, about 300g (10½oz), finely shredded
½ head of Chinese leaves, finely shredded
170g (6oz) bean sprouts
4 tbsp oyster sauce

Preparation time: 10 minutes
Cooking time: 4–6 minutes

1 Heat a small saucepan and dry-fry the sesame seeds, shaking the pan frequently, until they are just beginning to brown. Turn the seeds out into a small bowl and set aside.

2 Heat the oil in a wok or large frying pan. Add the onion and garlic, and stir-fry for 2–3 minutes or until softened slightly. Add the cabbage and Chinese leaves and stir-fry over a fairly high heat for 2–3 minutes or until the vegetables are just beginning to soften. Add the bean sprouts and continue cooking for a few seconds.

3 Make a space in the centre of the pan. Pour in the oyster sauce and 2 tbsp of water, and stir until hot, then toss the vegetables into the sauce. Taste and add pepper, with salt if necessary (this will depend on the saltiness of the oyster sauce). Serve at once, sprinkled with the toasted sesame seeds.

(V) **EACH SERVING PROVIDES:**
kcal 150, **protein** 5g, **fat** 11g (of which saturated fat 1g), **carbohydrate** 9g (of which sugars 5g), **fibre** 4g

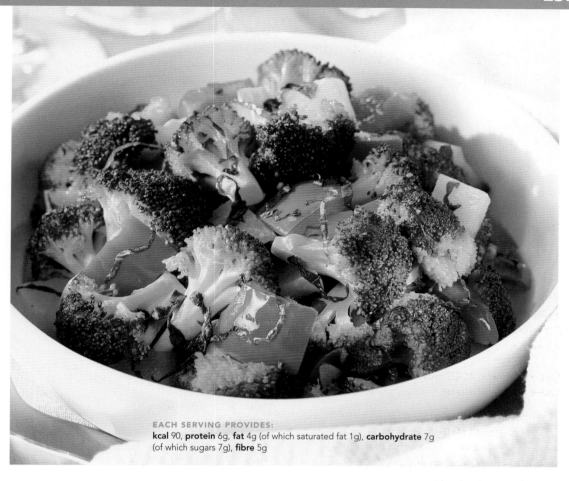

EACH SERVING PROVIDES:
kcal 90, **protein** 6g, **fat** 4g (of which saturated fat 1g), **carbohydrate** 7g
(of which sugars 7g), **fibre** 5g

Basil-scented sautéed vegetables

A large non-stick frying pan is ideal for sautéeing, a terrific method for preserving the colour of vegetables while bringing out their flavour to the full. Serve with fish, poultry or meat, or toss them with freshly cooked noodles.

Serves 4

500g (1lb 2oz) broccoli
1 tbsp extra virgin olive oil
3–4 large garlic cloves, thinly sliced (optional)
1 large or 2 small red peppers,
    seeded and cut into chunks
1 turnip, about 150g (5½oz), cut into bite-sized chunks
pinch of sugar
8 sprigs of fresh basil, stalks discarded,
    then finely shredded

Preparation time: 10 minutes
Cooking time: 7–8 minutes

1 Cut the broccoli into small florets; trim and thinly slice the stalks. Heat the olive oil in a large non-stick frying pan or wok. Add the garlic, if using, the red pepper, turnip and slices of broccoli stalk. Sprinkle in the sugar and salt to taste. Cook for 2–3 minutes, turning frequently.

2 Add the broccoli florets and stir. Pour in 6 tbsp of water to thinly coat the bottom of the pan. Cover and cook over a fairly high heat for 3–4 minutes. The broccoli should be just tender and bright green.

3 Stir in the basil, replace the lid and leave on the heat for a few more seconds. Serve immediately.

SNACKS

Piquant crab dip with crudités

This creamy dip is based on ingredients that can be kept in the storecupboard, so can be rustled up quickly if guests drop by unexpectedly. It is served with celery and cucumber sticks and pineapple wedges, all of which add important nutrients.

Serves 4
2 celery sticks, about 125g (4½oz) in total
½ cucumber, about 125g (4½oz)
1 small pineapple, about 340g (12oz)

CRAB DIP
1 can white crab meat, about 120g, drained
2 tbsp mayonnaise
2 tbsp plain low-fat yoghurt
1 tsp tomato purée
grated zest of 1 lime
30g (1oz) sun-dried tomatoes packed in oil, drained
        and finely chopped
30g (1oz) gherkins, finely chopped
a few drops of Tabasco sauce, or to taste

Preparation time: 15 minutes

1 To make the dip, put the crab meat, mayonnaise, yoghurt, tomato purée, lime zest, sun-dried tomatoes and gherkins in a bowl and stir together thoroughly. Season with Tabasco sauce to taste. Place the dip in a small serving bowl, cover and chill while preparing the crudités.

2 Cut the celery and cucumber into chunky sticks. Remove the crown of leaves from the pine-apple (wash and keep the leaves for garnish, if you like). Cut the flesh into wedges, leaving the skin on, then cut away the core.

3 Arrange the celery, cucumber and pineapple on a platter with the bowl of dip. Garnish with the pineapple leaves, if liked, and serve.

EACH SERVING
PROVIDES:
kcal 165, **protein** 8g, **fat** 10g (of which saturated fat 1g), **carbohydrate** 12g (of which sugars 11g), **fibre** 2g

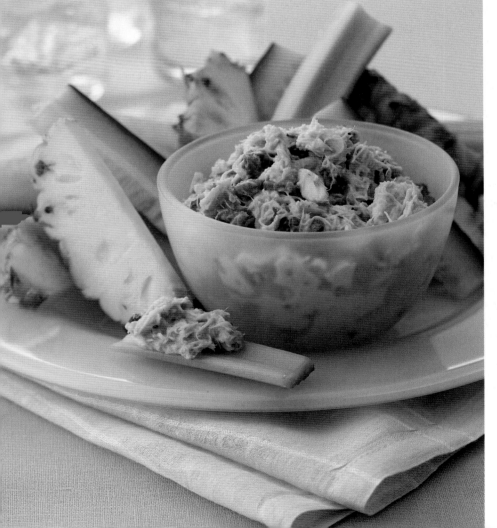

Ginger nuts

Here's a healthier, less fatty, version of a traditional favourite. You can prepare round biscuits, or buy some fancy cutters and encourage children to have a go at making gingerbread figures and shapes. Whatever the end result, these spicy, crunchy biscuits taste terrific.

Makes 12 biscuits

85g (3oz) plain white flour
85g (3oz) plain wholemeal flour
½ tsp bicarbonate of soda
2 tsp ground ginger
½ tsp ground cinnamon
50g (1¾oz) butter
4 tbsp golden syrup

Preparation time: 15 minutes
Cooking time: 8–10 minutes

1 Preheat the oven to 190°C (375°F, gas mark 5). Sift the white and wholemeal flours, bicarbonate of soda, ginger and cinnamon into a bowl, tipping in any bran left in the sieve.

2 Put the butter and golden syrup in a small pan and melt over a low heat, stirring occasionally. Pour the melted mixture onto the dry ingredients and stir to bind them together into a firm dough.

3 Break off a walnut-sized lump of dough and roll it into a ball on the palm of your hand. Press it flat into a thick biscuit, about 6cm (2½in) in diameter, and place on a greased baking sheet. Repeat with the remaining dough. (Or roll out the dough and stamp out decorative shapes.)

4 Bake the biscuits for 8–10 minutes or until they are slightly risen and browned. Leave to cool on the baking sheet for 2–3 minutes or until they are firm enough to lift without breaking, then transfer to a wire rack to cool completely. The biscuits can be kept in an airtight tin for up to 5 days.

EACH BISCUIT PROVIDES:
kcal 90, **protein** 1g, **fat** 4g (of which saturated fat 2g), **carbohydrate** 14g (of which sugars 4g), **fibre** 1g

Apple and muesli rock cakes

A little diced apple makes these rock cakes moist and fruity, and a perfect replacement for shop-bought biscuits. Easy to prepare, they are ideal to cook with younger members of the family, who will enjoy making these nutritious treats as much as eating them.

Makes 24 cakes

225g (8oz) self-raising flour
100g (3½oz) unsalted butter, cut into small pieces
55g (2oz) light muscovado sugar, plus a little
    extra to sprinkle
1 tsp ground cinnamon
2 dessert apples, peeled and diced
75g (2½oz) sugar-free muesli
1 egg, beaten
4–5 tbsp semi-skimmed milk, as needed

Preparation time: 20 minutes
Cooking time: 15 minutes

1 Preheat the oven to 190°C (375°F, gas mark 5). Put the flour into a bowl, add the butter and rub it in with your fingertips until the mixture resembles fine breadcrumbs.

2 Stir in the sugar, cinnamon, diced apples and muesli. Add the egg and stir it in with enough milk to bind the mixture together roughly.

3 Drop dessertspoonfuls of the mixture onto two greased baking sheets, leaving space around each cake, and sprinkle with a little extra sugar. Bake for 15 minutes or until golden and firm to the touch.

4 Transfer to a wire rack to cool, and serve warm or cold. The rock cakes can be kept in an airtight tin for up to 2 days.

EACH CAKE PROVIDES:
kcal 90, **protein** 2g, **fat** 4g (of which saturated fat 2g), **carbohydrate** 13g (of which sugars 4g), **fibre** 1g

Cereal bars

Naturally sweet and moist, these delicious bars will provide a great energy boost at any time of the day. They are also a good way of getting the family to try some more unusual grains and seeds, and adding new healthy ingredients to the diet.

Makes 14 bars

2 tbsp sunflower seeds
2 tbsp pumpkin seeds
2 tbsp linseeds
2 bananas, about 300g (10½oz) in total,
    weighed with their skins on
100g (3½oz) unsalted butter
3 tbsp golden syrup
50g (1¾oz) millet flakes
100g (3½oz) rolled oats
100g (3½oz) stoned dried dates,
    roughly chopped

Preparation time: 25 minutes
Cooking time: 30 minutes

1 Preheat the oven to 180°C (350°F, gas mark 4). Grease a 28 x 18 x 4cm (11 x 7 x 1½in) cake tin and line the bottom with baking parchment. Roughly chop the sunflower seeds, pumpkin seeds and linseeds. Peel and roughly mash the bananas.

2 Melt the butter in a saucepan and stir in the golden syrup. Add the chopped seeds and mashed bananas, together with the millet flakes, rolled oats and dates. Mix together well, then spoon the mixture into the prepared tin and level the surface.

3 Bake for about 30 minutes or until golden brown. Leave to cool in the tin for 5 minutes, then mark into 14 bars and leave to cool completely. The bars can be kept in an airtight tin for up to 2 days.

EACH BAR PROVIDES:
kcal 160, **protein** 3g, **fat** 10g (of which saturated fat 4g), **carbohydrate** 17g (of which sugars 8g), **fibre** 1g

Frozen pineapple and berry slush

A cross between a breakfast sorbet and a thick drink, this refreshing, virtually fat-free start to the day takes just seconds to whiz up. The secret of preparing it quickly is to keep a selection of chopped fruit in the freezer, then you can simply dip in to select a combination that suits your mood.

Serves 4

8 ice cubes
250g (9oz) hulled strawberries, frozen
250g (9oz) fresh pineapple chunks, frozen
120ml (4fl oz) pineapple juice
2 tbsp dried skimmed milk powder
1 tbsp vanilla sugar or caster sugar,
    or to taste
sprigs of fresh pineapple mint to decorate
    (optional)

Preparation time: 5–15 minutes, plus at least
    1½ hours freezing of fruit

1 Put the ice cubes in a food processor or heavy-duty blender and process until they are finely crushed. Alternatively, crush the ice cubes in a freezerproof bag, bashing them with a rolling pin, and then put them in the processor or blender.

2 Add the strawberries, pineapple chunks, pineapple juice and skimmed milk powder and process again until blended but still with small pieces of fruit and ice visible.

3 Taste and sweeten with sugar if necessary. (The amount of sugar required will depend on the sweetness of the fruit.) Process briefly using the pulse button.

4 Spoon into tall glasses, decorate each with a sprig of pineapple mint, if you like, and serve with long spoons.

EACH SERVING PROVIDES:
kcal 95, **protein** 3g, **fat** 0.3g, **carbohydrate** 22g (of which sugars 22g), **fibre** 2g

Summer pudding

What an amazing dish the British summer pudding is – delicious and simplicity itself. The peaches or nectarines add a slightly different dimension to this version – a great way of eating a large portion of ripe fresh uncooked fruit, which retains all its nutrients.

Serves 6

600g (1lb 5oz) mixed summer fruit
    (raspberries, blueberries, redcurrants,
    sliced strawberries)
2 ripe peaches or nectarines, stoned and diced
3 tbsp sugar, or to taste
150ml (5fl oz) cranberry juice
8 thin slices white bread, about
    200g (7oz) in total, preferably
    1–2 days old
TO SERVE (optional)
reduced-fat crème fraîche

Preparation time: 20 minutes,
    plus 2 hours macerating
    and 8 hours chilling

1 Crush the different types of fruit individually, to be sure all the skins are broken and the fruit is pulpy. Put all the fruit in a large bowl with the sugar and cranberry juice and stir to mix. Leave to macerate for 2 hours.

2 Cut the crusts from the bread and cut the slices into strips or triangles. Fit the bread into a 1 litre (2 pint) pudding basin to line the bottom and sides, reserving enough bread to cover the top. Fill in any gaps with small bits of bread.

3 Reserve 3–4 tbsp of juice from the mixed fruit, then gently pour the fruit mixture into the bread-lined pudding basin. Top with the remaining bread. Cover with a plate that just fits inside the rim of the basin, setting it directly on top of the bread, then place a heavy weight such as a can of food on top. Place in the fridge to chill for 8 hours or overnight.

4 To serve, turn the pudding out onto a serving dish. Use the reserved fruit juice to brush or pour over any parts of the bread that have not been coloured. Serve with crème fraîche, if liked.

EACH SERVING (PUDDING ALONE) PROVIDES:
kcal 160, **protein** 4g, **fat** 1g, **carbohydrate** 36g
(of which sugars 20g), **fibre** 3g

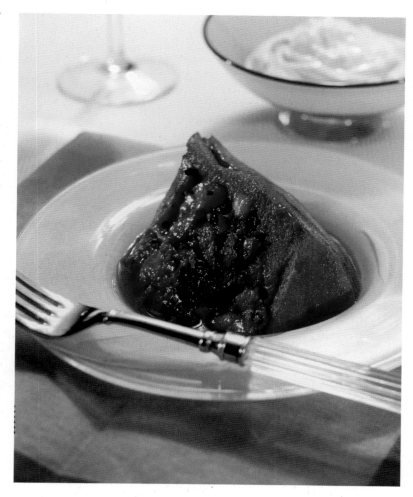

Rich chocolate torte

A generous amount of good-quality dark chocolate makes this Continental-style cake moist and rich – just a small slice will satisfy any sweet tooth. It's perfect as a warm dessert, with a spoonful of soured cream or Greek-style yoghurt and some fresh berries.

Serves 10

170g (6oz) good dark chocolate (at least
    70% cocoa solids)
75g (2½oz) unsalted butter
4 eggs
100g (3½oz) light muscovado sugar
30g (1oz) plain flour
TO DECORATE
Cape gooseberries, papery skins folded back
    (optional)
icing sugar and cocoa powder

Preparation time: 20 minutes
Cooking time: 15–20 minutes

1 Preheat the oven to 180°C (350°F, gas mark 4). Grease a 23cm (9in) springform cake tin and line it with greased greaseproof paper.

2 Break up the chocolate and put it in a heatproof bowl with the butter. Set the bowl over a pan of almost boiling water, making sure that the water is not touching the base of the bowl. Leave the chocolate and butter to melt, then remove from the heat and stir the mixture until smooth.

3 Meanwhile, put the eggs and sugar in a large bowl and beat with an electric mixer until the mixture has increased considerably in volume and leaves a trail on the surface when the beaters are lifted out. (If using a hand whisk or rotary beater, set the bowl over a pan of almost boiling water, making sure the water is not touching the base of the bowl.)

4 Add the chocolate mixture to the whisked mixture and fold it in with a large metal spoon. Gradually sift the flour over the top of the egg and chocolate mixture, folding in until it is just combined.

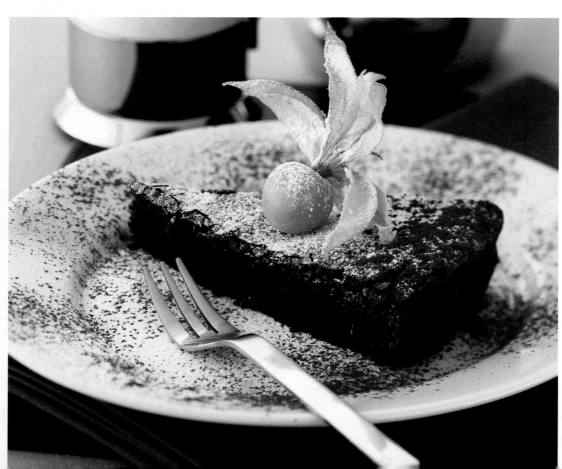

5 Turn the mixture into the prepared cake tin and gently spread it to the edges to level the surface. Bake for 15–20 minutes or until the top of the cake feels just firm to the touch. Leave to cool in the tin.

6 Take the cake from the tin and peel away the lining paper. Serve in thin wedges, decorating each with a Cape gooseberry, if liked, and dusting the plates with sifted icing sugar and cocoa powder. The cake can be kept in the fridge for 2–3 days.

EACH SERVING PROVIDES:
kcal 230, **protein** 4g, **fat** 14g (of which saturated fat 8g), **carbohydrate** 24g (of which sugars 21g), **fibre** 0g

Pannacotta

The traditional recipe for this 'cooked cream', from the Piedmont region of Italy, is made with rich double cream. This lighter version, served with a pretty fruit compote, is still smooth and creamy yet much lower in fat. Prepare it the day before serving, if possible.

Serves 4

500ml (17fl oz) semi-skimmed milk
1 tbsp powdered gelatine
75g (2½oz) caster sugar
100ml (3½fl oz) single cream
strip of pared orange zest
1 vanilla pod, split
RHUBARB AND STRAWBERRY COMPOTE
400g (14oz) pink rhubarb, trimmed and cut
        into 5cm (2in) lengths
juice of 1 orange
30g (1oz) caster sugar
450g (1lb) ripe strawberries, sliced

**Preparation and cooking time: 30 minutes,
        plus at least 3 hours chilling**

1 Pour 150ml (5fl oz) of the milk into a saucepan. Sprinkle over the gelatine and leave to soak, without stirring, for 5 minutes or until the gelatine has become spongy.

2 Stir in the sugar, then set the pan over a low heat. Warm gently, without boiling, until the gelatine and sugar have completely dissolved, stirring frequently.

3 Remove the pan from the heat and add the remaining milk, the cream and orange zest. Scrape the seeds from the vanilla pod into the milk mixture, then add the pod too. Leave to infuse for 10 minutes while preparing the compote.

4 Place the rhubarb in a saucepan with the orange juice and sugar. Bring just to a simmer, then cook gently for 3–4 minutes or until the rhubarb is tender but still holding its shape. Spoon the rhubarb into a serving dish using a draining spoon. Boil the juice remaining in the pan to reduce it slightly until syrupy. Pour the juice over the rhubarb and gently stir in the sliced strawberries. Leave to cool.

5 Strain the milk mixture through a fine sieve into a jug, then pour into 4 moulds, cups or ramekins of 170ml (6fl oz) capacity. Allow to cool, then cover and chill for at least 3 hours or until set.

6 To serve, run the tip of a knife around the edge of each pannacotta. Place an inverted serving plate over the top of the ramekin and turn them upside down, holding the two firmly together. Lift off the ramekin. Spoon some of the compote on the side of the pannacotta. Serve the remaining compote separately.

EACH SERVING PROVIDES:
kcal 265, **protein** 10g, **fat** 7g (of which saturated fat 4g), **carbohydrate** 43g (of which sugars 43g), **fibre** 3g

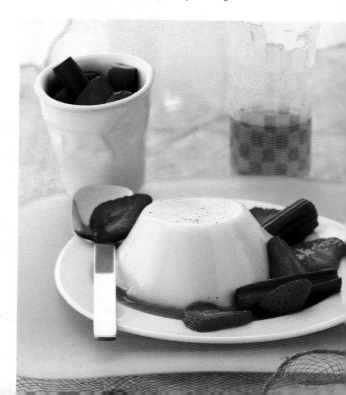

INDEX

A

AbioCor 207
ACE (angiotensin-converting enzyme) 185
ACE (angiotensin-converting enzyme)
  inhibitors 180, 181
Actilyse 184
activity log 109, 123, 134, 137, 146
acupuncture
  for heart failure 209
  for smoking cessation 63
Adalat 183
adipose (fatty) tissue 130
adrenaline 151
Advil 184
aerobic exercise 103-4, 107, 121
age
  and bypass surgery 194
  and exercise 119
  and heart disease 19, 21, 26
Aggrastat 185
alcohol 92-94
  benefits 92-93, 94
  health risks 94
  and liver disease 93, 94
  and mental acuity 93
  moderate consumption 92
  wine 93
alcoholism 44, 94
alpha-beta-blockers 180
alpha-blockers 180
alteplase 184
Alzheimer's disease 84
Amias 181
amlodipine 183
anaemia 202

anger
  and heart disease 16, 151, 154, 155, 157
  management 160, 161
angina 40, 41, 48, 62
  and angioplasty 195, 196
  and bypass surgery 193, 194
  case histories 57, 156
  enhanced external counterpulsation (EECP)
    201-2
  exertional angina 41, 57
  and HRT 172
  medication 181-3, 185, 194
  men/women 165, 167
  stress and 152
  symptoms 40
  transmyocardial revascularization (TMR) 201
  unstable angina 41, 185, 194
angiogram 48, 53, 54-55, 57, 167
angioplasty 47, 57, 195-6, 198-200, 208
  and bypass surgery compared 196, 201
  coronary brachytherapy 199
  embolization protection devices 198
  heart attack risk 196
  laser angioplasty 200
  photoangioplasty 198, 200
  restenosis 198-200, 208
  statistics 199
  stents 57, 199-200, 201, 208
angiotensin receptor blockers (ARBs) 180-1
anticoagulants 184-5
antioxidants 84, 87, 89, 96, 97, 99, 179
  and statin drugs 179
appetite suppressants 142
Apresoline 181
Aprovel 181
arginine 87
arrhythmias 44, 45, 48, 51, 79, 94, 120,
  180, 204
arteriosclerosis 35
artificial hearts 191, 207
aspirin 40, 42, 177, 183-4, 185
  super aspirins 177, 185
atenolol 180
atherectomy 196
atherosclerosis 13, 17, 18, 21, 29, 39,
  42, 89, 211
  smoking and 30
atorvastatin 178, 179
automatic external defibrillators (AEDs) 42
avocados 89-90

B

bacterial infections 35
basic fibroblast growth factor 195
bendroflumethiazide 180
beta-blockers 120, 180, 183
beta carotene 96
beta-sitosterol 89
Betaloc 180
bile acid sequestrants 179
bionic heart 207
blood clots 40, 94
  alcohol and 93
  anticoagulants 184-5
  dissolving 165, 184-5
  embolism 196, 208
  formation 14, 27, 39, 41-42, 151, 152, 157
  HPA-2 Met gene 35
  prevention 75, 78, 89
  smoking and 61
  stress and 151, 152
blood flow 48
blood pressure
  decongestants and 183
  diastolic blood pressure 24, 28, 180
  high see hypertension
  home monitors 25
  lowering 121, 163, 180-1, 182
  measuring 27, 47
  optimal 26, 28
  and smoking 61
  systolic blood pressure 24, 28
blood sugar levels 91, 92, 140
blood tests 48-49
blood transfusions 202
body fat 31
body mass index (BMI) 24, 99, 131
body shape 31
boredom 220
Borg Perceived Exertion Scale 120
bread 92, 98
breakfasts 92
  recipes 223-4
breast cancer 89, 94, 167
  alcohol and 94
  HRT and 172, 173, 174
  soya, benefits of 89
breath, shortness of 40, 42, 169

breathing
  breathing exercises 71
  and heart defects 48
  in meditation 163
British Heart Foundation 220
British Regional Heart Study 102
bronchitis 40, 61
bruit 48
buddy systems 218-20
bupropion 62, 64
bypass surgery see coronary bypass surgery

C

Calciparine 185
calcium-channel blockers 180, 182-3
calories 99
  burning 122, 127, 130, 136, 146-7, 149
  calorie counter 134
  cutting 138, 139-41, 143
  high-volume low-calorie foods 140-1
  low-calorie menu 144
  and weight-loss diets 138-9
cancer
  breast cancer 89, 94, 167, 172, 173, 174
  colon cancer 94
  lung cancer 61, 96
  prostate cancer 89
candesartan 181
Capoten 180
captopril 180
carbohydrates 91, 99
  complex carbohydrates 91, 92, 140
  low-fat high-carbohydrate diet 36, 77, 78
  simple (refined) carbohydrates 91, 140, 170
carbon monoxide 14, 30
cardiac enzymes 48, 49
cardiomyopathy 45, 48
cardiovascular disease 11, 18
  age and 19
  mortality rates 11, 13
  numbers affected 11
Cardura 180
carotid artery disease 13, 18, 39
carotid phonoangiogram 53
cereals 90, 92, 98
cerivastatin 178
chest pain 40, 41, 42, 102, 152, 156, 169, 212
chest pressure/tightness 40, 41, 42, 169

D

dairy spreads 79
death
  falling death rates 11, 12, 13
  heart attacks 13, 42, 45, 167
  top five causes 16
  women 166-7
decongestants 183
defibrillators 42, 48, 206
depression 151, 157
  exercise, benefits of 161
  post-operative depression 193, 203
  and risk of heart disease 157
  symptoms 157
dessert recipes 241-3
diabetes 15, 23, 29
  family medical history 25
  risk factor for heart disease 23-24, 29, 91, 168
  risk reduction 101, 103, 127, 170
  Type 1 diabetes 29
  Type 2 (adult-onset) diabetes 29, 85, 91, 103, 127
  weight factor 16, 31, 127
  women and 168, 170
diagnosis 38-57
  physical examination 47-48
  see also **diagnostic tests**
diagnostic tests
  angiography 48, 53, 54-55, 57, 167
  blood tests 48-49
  chest X-ray 52-53
  computed tomography (CT) 53, 55, 56
  echocardiography 55
  electrocardiogram 48, 49-51
  electrophysiologic tests 51
  magnetic resonance imaging (MRI) 53, 55, 56
  positron emission tomography (PET) 55, 56
  radioisotope scanning 48, 53-54
diastolic blood pressure 24, 28, 180
diet 13, 14, 16, 72-99
  alcohol 92-94
  antioxidants 84
  blood sugar levels 91-92
  calorie counting 99
  changing 18-21, 98-99
  crash diets 132
  fat content 34
  food diary 218

  fruit and vegetables 84, 86, 98, 99, 138, 139, 143, 146
  healthy diet 73-74
  high-protein diet 36, 132
  low-fat diet 36, 80, 143
  low-fat high-carbohydrate diet 36, 77, 78
  Mediterranean diet 80, 81
  nutrient-dense foods 140
  portion sizes 139
  processed foods 14, 90-91, 95
  pub and restaurant food 88
  quiz 76-77
  rehabilitation period 212
  salt consumption 95
  seasonal food 80
  superstar foods 87, 89-90
  vitamin supplements 35, 96-98
  vs medication 182
  weight-loss plans 131-2
  whole-grain foods 90, 92, 98, 99, 170
  see also **cholesterol**; **fats**; **fibre**; **weight, losing**
diltiazem 183
dinner recipes 230-5
diuretics 180
doxazosin 180
drug abuse 44
drug therapies *see* **medication**

E

ECG *see* **electrocardiogram**
echocardiogram 48
echocardiography 48, 55
eggs 83
electrocardiogram (ECG) 48, 49-51
  ambulatory ECG 50-1
  exercise ECG (stress test) 48, 49-50
  resting ECG 49
electroencephalogram (EEG) 53
electrophysiologic tests 51
embolism 196, 208
embolization protection devices 198
emotions, negative 16, 151, 154-5, 157
emphysema 40, 61
enalapril 180
endorphins 123
endothelin-1 93
enhanced external counterpulsation (EECP) 201-2

and heart failure 202, 204
medications 12, 180-1
risk factor for heart disease 23-24, 26-27, 32, 36, 168-169
salt consumption and 95
and sleep apnoea 44
stress and 152
and stroke 15
and Syndrome X 36
and weight 16, 127, 130, 170
'white coat' hypertension 25
women 168-9
hyperthyroidism 129
hypnotherapy 63
hypothyroidism 129, 130
Hypovase 180
Hytrin 180

I, J

ibuprofen 184
immune system, boosting 107
impotence 62, 64
Inderal 180
inflammation 35, 43, 45, 49
  anti-inflammatory foods 79
Innovace 180
insulin 29, 85, 91, 92
insulin resistance 36
InSync Biventricular Cardiac Pacing System 204
irbesartan 181
ischaemia 41, 44, 560
  myocardial ischaemia 41, 48
  silent ischaemia 48
Istin 183
Jarvik 206
Jarvik 2000 Heart 206

L

labetalol 180
lactate dehydrogenase 49
laser angioplasty 200
laughter, benefits of 151, 162
lentils 87
Lescol 179
lifestyle 211, 215

risk factors for heart disease 24, 30-32
sedentary lifestyle 14, 31-32, 101-2, 216
lifestyle changes 14, 16-18, 182, 211, 215-21
  buddy systems 218-20
  goals 218, 219
  stages of change 17-21
  strategies 216, 218-21
  willpower 217
Lifestyle Heart Trial 80
LifeVest 206
lipid clinics 43
Lipitor 178, 179
Lipobay 178
lipoproteins 35
Lipostat 179
lisinopril 180
Loniten 181
losartan 181
low-fat diet 36, 80, 143
low-fat high-carbohydrate diet 36, 77, 78
Lp(a) 35
lung cancer 61, 96
Lyon Diet Heart Study 81

M

magnetic resonance imaging (MRI) 53, 55, 56
  'black blood MRI' 51
  ultrafast MRI 55
meat 98
medication 176-89
  angina 181-3, 185
  anticoagulants 184-5
  aspirin therapy 40, 42, 177, 183-4, 185
  blood pressure medications 180-1
  cholesterol-lowering drugs 12, 43, 177, 178-80, 186
  coronary artery disease 181-5
  heart attacks 183-5
  noncompliance 185-7
  pill organizers 188, 189
  prescription errors 187
  reminders 188-9
  side effects 187
  vs bypass surgery 194
  vs diet 182
meditation 163
Mediterranean diet 16, 80, 81

protein 138

pumps *see* **ventricular assist devices**

quality of life 213

Questran 179

R

radioisotope scanning 48, 53-54
  single photon emission computed tomography (SPECT) 54

raloxifene 173

rapeseed oil 79

recipes 222-43
  breakfast 223-4
  desserts 241-3
  dinners 230-5
  salads 224-6
  sandwiches 226-7
  snacks 238-40
  soups 228-9
  vegetables 235-7

rehabilitation 203, 211, 212
  case histories 197, 214
  diet 212
  exercise 211-12
  lifestyle changes 215-21
  relaxation 213-14

relaxation 16, 159, 162-3, 203, 213-14

resistance training (strength training) 103

restaurant food 88

restenosis 198-200, 208

resting heart rate 47

resting metabolic rate (RMR) 130

rhabdomyolysis 178

rice 90, 91, 92, 99

risk factors 20, 22-37
  age 23, 26
  bacterial and viral infections 35
  C-reactive protein 35, 43
  cholesterol 20, 25, 29, 169
  combinations 32, 36
  cultural difference 23
  depression 157
  diabetes 23-24, 29, 91, 168
  family medical history 20, 23, 25
  gender factors 23, 25-26, 165-7
  high cholesterol levels 23, 25, 29, 169
  homocysteine levels 35
  HPA-2 Met 35

hypertension 23-24, 26-27, 32, 36, 168-9
  inflammation 35
  lifestyle factors 24, 30-32
  lipoproteins 35
  myths about 20
  negative emotions 16, 151, 154-5, 157
  obesity 30-31, 171-2
  oral contraceptives 171
  quiz (personal assessment) 33
  risk reduction 20, 21, 24, 26-32, 34, 37, 86
  sedentary lifestyle 14, 31-32, 101-2, 171-2
  sleep apnoea 44
  smoking 30, 32, 169
  stress 151, 152
  Syndrome X 36
  Type A personality 154-5

rosuvastatin 179

S, T

salads 224-6

salt 95

sandwich recipes 226-7

saphenous vein 192

saturated fats 11, 12, 21, 34, 74, 75, 76, 78, 80, 81, 83, 99, 132, 140

Scottish Heart Health Study 87

sedentary lifestyle 14, 31-32, 101-2, 216
  risk factor for heart disease 14, 31-32, 102, 171
  women 171

selective oestrogen receptor modulators (SERMs) 173

self-confidence 121

Seven Countries Study 23, 79

sexual function 212
  impotence 62, 64

silent ischaemia 48

simvastatin 178, 179

single photon emission computed tomography (SPECT) 54

sleep apnoea 44

Slow Food movement 141

smoking 32, 58-71, 211
  addiction 59-60
  and blood pressure 61
  and cholesterol 61
  cigar smokers 61
  cravings 67

CREDITS

COVER PhotoDisc. **2–3** PhotoDisc. **5** EyeWire. **7** ImageState. **8** TOP TO BOTTOM Brand X Pictures, PhotoSpin, Brand X Pictures, Brand X Pictures, ImageState, PhotoDisc. **9** TOP TO BOTTOM Comstock, PhotoDisc, EyeWire, PhotoDisc, PhotoDisc, Corbis. **10** Brand X Pictures. **12** PhotoDisc. **15** Brand X Pictures. **16** PhotoDisc. **17** ImageState. **18** CSA Images. **19** PhotoDisc. **20** EyeWire. **21** Comstock. **22** PhotoSpin. **25** PhotoSpin. **26** PhotoDisc. **27** CSA Images. **28** Comstock. **31** LEFT Corbis, RIGHT Artville. **32** PhotoDisc. **33** Brand X Pictures. **34** EyeWire. **35** CSA Images. **37** LEFT DigitalVision/PictureQuest, RIGHT PhotoDisc. **38** Brand X Pictures. **40** DigitalVision/PictureQuest. **41** PhotoDisc. **43** PhotoDisc. **44** Brand X Pictures. **46** PhotoDisc. **47** PhotoDisc. **49** PhotoDisc. **50** Brand X Pictures. **52** PhotoDisc. **53** PhotoSpin. **54** ISM/Phototake. **57** Brand X Pictures. **58** Brand X Pictures. **60** Ray Laskowitz/Brand X Pictures/PictureQuest. **63** PhotoDisc. **64** PhotoDisc. **65** Brand X Pictures. **67** PhotoDisc. **69** TOP Corbis, BOTTOM PhotoDisc. **70** ImageState. **72** ImageState. **75** PhotoDisc. **77** ALL PhotoDisc. **78** PhotoSpin. **80** Artville. **81** Comstock. **82** PhotoDisc. **83** Corbis. **84** Artville. **85** ImageState. **86** TOP PhotoDisc, CENTRE AND BOTTOM Artville. **88** PhotoSpin. **89** PhotoDisc. **90** EyeWire. **91** PhotoDisc. **92** Brand X Pictures. **94** Artville. **95** Corbis. **96** Reader's Digest Assoc./GID. **98** PhotoDisc. **100** PhotoDisc. **102** Comstock. **103** PhotoSpin. **104** ImageState. **106** Julie Johnson. **107** PhotoDisc. **108** Comstock. **110** PhotoSpin. **111** John Nietzel. **112** PhotoSpin. **113** PhotoSpin. **115** PhotoDisc. **116–117** Julie Johnson. **119** DigitalVision/PictureQuest. **122** LEFT PhotoDisc, MIDDLE PhotoSpin, RIGHT PhotoDisc. **123** PhotoSpin. **124** Stockbyte/PictureQuest. **126** Comstock. **131** EyeWire. **133** PhotoDisc. **134** EyeWire. **138** PhotoSpin. **139** EyeWire. **140** PhotoDisc. **141** Reader's Digest Assoc./GID. **143** Reader's Digest Assoc./GID. **144** TOP PhotoDisc, CENTER PhotoSpin, BOTTOM Reader's Digest Assoc./GID. **148** PhotoDisc. **149** PhotoDisc. **150** PhotoDisc. **152** ImageState. **153** ImageState **154** PhotoDisc. **156** PhotoDisc. **157** InterCure, Inc. **158** PhotoDisc. **159** Reader's Digest Assoc./GID. **160** ImageState. **161** PhotoDisc. **162** ImageState. **163** Corbis. **164** EyeWire. **168** Comstock. **170** EyeWire. **171** EyeWire. **175** Comstock. **176** PhotoDisc. **179** Reader's Digest Assoc./GID. **180** PhotoDisc. **183** PhotoSpin. **187** EyeWire. **188** PhotoDisc. **189** MEDport. **190** PhotoDisc. **194** Comstock. **196** Reader's Digest Assoc./GID. **197** Brand X Pictures. **199** Medtronic, Inc. **202** PhotoDisc **204** Medtronic, Inc. **205** FischerHealth, Inc. **206** LIFECOR, Inc. **207** ABIOMED, Inc. **209** Corbis. **210** Corbis. **213** EyeWire. **215** PhotoDisc. **219** PhotoDisc. **221** RubberBall Productions. **223–243** Reader's Digest Association Ltd.

ISBN 0 276 44043 9
Book code 400-248-01
Oracle code 250006197H.00.24